Praise for **Recovering fro**

"Todd has done an excellent job of providing a thorough, concise and balanced understanding of emotional trauma and what healing needs to include. It provides an understanding of the deep, underlying issues, as well as an understanding of practical tools for healing - both the deeper issues as well as responding in the present when our emotional wounds are triggered. One quickly realizes that Todd is not just giving us academic information from a remote ivory tower; he has walked this journey of healing in his own life. This is advice that comes from scientific research and personal experience."

- **Tim Fletcher**, Founder and President of RE/ACT, trauma educator, YouTuber, and host of the *Time with Tim Fletcher* podcast.

"In your hands you hold a blueprint to the life you want. Dr. Todd provides a way you can navigate your past, move through your present, and create your future in a way you might not have even imagined. It will never be easy, and your road will be filled with speed bumps, potholes, and even another sinkhole of sorts. Keep this book within arm's reach and refer to it often. It is filled with practical steps you can take to reconnect to what matters most in your life or work. It will touch your heart, strengthen your resolve, and fill your days with moments of hope you can hang on to during your road to recovery, and possibility."

- **Mark LeBlanc**, CSP, CPAE, author of *Never Be the Same*

"If you've ever felt broken, unseen, or unsure of who you truly are, this book is a lifeline. He is a gifted writer with a rare ability to blend lived experience and clinical wisdom. The holistic healing approach he brilliantly lays out will help you navigate your healing journey with much more clarity and purpose."

- **Dannie Reeve**, Bioneuroemotion practitioner, coach, writer, and co-host of the *Happy Neurotics* podcast.

RECOVERING
—— FROM ——
EMOTIONAL TRAUMA

Essential Tools to Calm Your Emotions,
Heal Your Sense of Self, and Strengthen Relationships

TODD BERNTSON

DTI Publishing
Saint Paul, MN

Recovering from Emotional Trauma

©2026 Todd Berntson

Printed in the United States of America. All rights reserved. No part of this book may be reproduced or transmitted in any form or by any means, electronic or mechanical, including photocopying, recording, or by any information storage and retrieval system, without written permission from the author.

The information provided within this book is for general entertainment and informational purposes only. This work depicts actual events, locales, and conversations as truthfully as possible, recalled from personal memories.

Although every effort has been made to ensure that information in this book was correct at press time, the author does not assume, and hereby disclaims, any liability to any party for any loss, damage, or disruption caused by errors or omissions, whether such errors or omissions result from negligence, accident, or any other cause. Some names have been changed to protect privacy.

NO AI TRAINING: Without in any way limiting the author's and publisher's exclusive rights under copyright, any use of this publication to "train" generative artificial intelligence (AI) technologies to generate text is expressly prohibited. The author reserves all rights to license uses of this work for generative AI training and development of machine learning language models.

Ordering Information:
Quantity sales. Special discounts are available on quantity purchases by corporations, associations, and others.

Library of Congress Control Number: 2025916138

DTI Publishing
St. Paul, MN

Cover images #347850190 and #1165853579 licensed under Adobe Stock Extended License.

ISBN (Hardcover): 979-8-9926061-0-2
ISBN (Paperback): 979-8-9926061-1-9

Dedication to all of the people who helped me in my own recovery. I could not have done it without you!

Contents

Chapter 1: Emerging from the Darkness 1
Chapter 2: What Is Emotional Trauma? 15
Chapter 3: Our Dysregulated Emotions 39
Chapter 4: Our Damaged Self-Concept 63
Chapter 5: Our Difficulties with Relationships 89
Chapter 6: The Holistic Healing Mindset 115
Chapter 7: Calming Your Emotions 129
Chapter 8: Healing Your Core Self-Concept 155
Chapter 9: Strenthening Your Relationships 177
Chapter 10: Your Journey of Recovery 201
Resources 217
Index 219
Acknowledgments 223
About the Author 225

CHAPTER 1

Emerging from the Darkness

IF YOU ARE READING this book, chances are good that you are living with the effects of some hurtful past experience and are looking for some help. Well, you have come to the right place. In the following pages, you will learn how certain kinds of stressful experience changes the way your brain processes emotion, affects the development of your core sense of self, and impacts the way you relate to others. You will learn a holistic approach to healing that will help you recover from the effects of emotional trauma so that you can live the life that you want.

It is important to know that you are not a broken or flawed human being who has no hope of recovery. If you experienced emotional trauma, you are simply living with the effects of an emotional injury. Those injuries can be healed. As a therapist who has helped many people recover from emotional trauma, and as someone who has lived its effects myself, I know first-hand how distressing emotional trauma can be.

My Story

In 1988, I was a student at Minneapolis Community College taking general education classes in the hopes of one day getting a bachelor's degree. I had no idea what I wanted to do, but I figured that going to college would help me get there—wherever that was. As I was meandering down the main hallway one day, I saw a poster announcing that the Sexual Violence Center of Minneapolis was looking for volunteer counselors. For reasons that I didn't understand at the time, that poster stirred something in me, so I decided to sign up for their training program.

The topic of one of the classes was about male victims of sexual abuse. I remember feeling surprised by the idea that sexual assault also happened to boys and men. Like many people at the time, I had assumed that it only happened to girls and women. As the trainer went through his presentation, however, I felt as though he was describing my experience. Every word seemed to resonate with me. At one point, he listed the common symptoms seen in adult men who had experienced sexual trauma as children, such as dissociation, addiction, difficulty urinating in public restrooms, precocious hypersexuality, depression, and a few others. I sat there stunned. I had every single one of the symptoms he listed—and to a significant degree. Then a sense of heaviness came over me.

- Had I experienced sexual abuse?
- If so, why can't I remember?
- Was I drawn to be here because this had happened to me?
- Am I just imagining this, or was I really abused?

For days afterward, I tried to recall what may have happened to me. What kept coming up was a nagging sense that something occurred at a school that I had attended when I was about five years old.

Abuse at the School

I don't remember much about it, only flashes of memory that seem bizarre and disjointed. I remember hiding under a car in the parking lot while someone was trying to find me. I remember being in a dark hallway in the basement. I remember feelings of being trapped and panicking. Aside from those flashes, I had no memory at all.

I called my mom to ask her about the school and whether something happened to me there. As soon as I brought it up, she began to nervously clear her throat and seemed to choose her words carefully. I could tell that she knew something she didn't want to share, which was typical of her "let's smile and pretend that nothing bad is happening" way of parenting. The most I was able to get out of her was that she finally decided to pull me out of the school one day after I shook and screamed so violently when she tried to drop me off that she had to take me back home.

There is a part of me that wishes I could remember what happened at that school. If I could, then I could point to it and say, "See! That's why I was so messed up!" But my experience at that school is merely a jumble of sensations, images, and feelings. While the emotional consequences of the experience still live within me, any detail about what actually occurred was never encoded into any coherent memory. There are bits and pieces, but nothing that makes sense.

I have since come to understand that a lack of memory of a traumatic event is common with childhood sexual abuse. The details about what happened probably don't matter all that much. Remembering wouldn't change the damage that was done to my sense of self, it wouldn't reduce the impact that the trauma had on the emotional circuits in my brain, and it wouldn't make healing any easier.

The events from that school are not the only reason why I struggled with a broken sense of self as an adult. At the time,

I certainly had the typical childhood symptoms of abuse, such as night terrors, wetting the bed, unexplained constipation, and starting fires, but it was only part of the story. Growing up in a home with parents who were alcoholic, were emotionally absent, and had been traumatized themselves also played a significant role in my disrupted sense of self.

Children rarely recognize that they are being emotionally harmed when they are young because they don't know any different. If you were to ask me about my family life when I was ten years old, I would tell you what a wonderful family I had. I was a typical kid who idolized my parents and had no idea that I was growing up in an unhealthy environment. Like most people who have been negatively impacted by their childhood, it wasn't until adulthood that the effects of my experience began to emerge.

Unfortunately, the experiences of my childhood resulted in my entering into adulthood as a depressed, disoriented, and suicidal human being. By the time I was eighteen years old, I was an addict who lived in an abandoned house and was literally using drugs to die. I was so dissociated from my emotions that I often bragged about not having any emotion at all. The reality was quite different. My internal world was seething with feelings of hurt, worthlessness, emptiness, anger, disorientation, and self-hatred. Marijuana, alcohol, and LSD were the only things that gave me a reprieve from having to feel, and at the time, I would rather have died than feel something. Living with the effects of emotional trauma had brought me to a very dark place, and I was just done. I felt like life had blown a hole through my soul, and carrying around the emptiness and pain had worn me down to the point where I didn't want to live anymore. I was profoundly depressed and felt alone and helpless. I wanted it all to end.

The Day Everything Changed

It was about 2:30 in the morning on September 10, 1983, and I was standing in the kitchen of the abandoned house. I suddenly felt my body freeze in place and I was surrounded by a pale yellow light. Everything in the room seemed different. It was as though the room had expanded by about twenty feet in all directions, and nothing had any color other than the yellow hue from the light that enveloped me. I didn't feel scared. If anything, I felt a sense of calm. After a moment, I heard a resounding voice say "You don't have to live like this anymore." Then it was all over.

Some people have asked me whether I thought it was an acid flashback, others have asked if I thought it was God intervening in my life, and some just don't believe me when I tell this part of my story. Having experienced acid flashbacks, I can say with certainty that it wasn't that. I wasn't even high at the time it happened. Was I touched by God? I honestly don't know. All I know is that the experience was real, and it caused a fundamental reorientation in my life. What I didn't realize at the time was that although I had gone to that house to die, what I had been gifted was an opportunity for a new life, if I was willing to put in the work. That was over 40 years ago, and thanks to becoming involved in a 12-Step Program, I have been completely clean of all alcohol and drugs ever since.

My Journey Through Insanity

I wish I could say that the moment I became sober, my life was suddenly happy, joyous, and free. But that was not the case. I was an utter emotional and psychological wreck, and I no longer had drugs and alcohol to numb the emptiness and pain. Every day, I felt myself being thrown around by a chaotic storm of intense emotions and racing thoughts that I didn't understand. I would cycle through periods of effusive enthusiastic optimism, and then become flooded with intense feelings of worthlessness, isolation, rage, and despair. It seemed that everything in my life was further evidence of how much of a loser I was and how everyone hated me.

I carried an intense emptiness within me, and I longed to be seen, to be loved, to be accepted, and to feel valued. This frequently led to people-pleasing behavior where I would give away everything to others in an effort to get them to see me as valuable. I felt a hole in my soul that never seemed to go away, no matter what I did, how many therapists I saw, or how many affirmations I recited to myself in the mirror. Life felt like a constant struggle to find a place where I felt safe and wanted.

I had an almost constant sense of urgency to rush somewhere else or to start something new in a desperate effort to "finally find myself." I impulsively bought things I couldn't afford, abruptly ended relationships with people I loved, struggled to maintain a job, and literally could not sit still. Despite my best attempts at approximating normal behavior, the dysregulated state of my emotions drove me to act in ways that were unpredictable and at times, bizarre. In fact, during one particularly intense episode of ill-defined panic, I took the front seats out of my car and threw them into a dumpster. It never occurred to me what a weird thing that was to do. For the next year, I sat on a milk crate whenever I had to drive.

Emotional flashbacks of intense violent imagery flooded me on an almost daily basis. I still recall one instance where I walked out of a bookstore and was suddenly consumed by a vision of a man rushing up to me and violently stabbing me in the chest over and over again. I stood there for a moment in a state of shock. The violent emotional flashback subsided after a few minutes, and I realized that it was just "another one of those terrifying things" that had become a normal part of my day.

During this whole time, I recognized that something about me was not normal, but I couldn't figure out what it was. What appeared to be so easy for other people was hard or impossible for me. Although I had been sober for quite a few years and was doing well in my recovery from addiction, the effects of untreated emotional trauma continued to erode my sense of self. I was afraid to open up to others and share what I was experiencing because it seemed that every time I did, people looked at me like I was crazy. I felt that if people really knew who I was, they would reject me. So, I developed a convincing presentation of normalcy to keep everyone from knowing the real person behind the shiny facade.

Emerging from the Darkness

Recovering from emotional trauma was neither quick nor easy for me. It has taken me a many years to get to the semi-sane state that I am in today. A hard truth that I have come to understand is that emotional trauma is very difficult to treat. While many therapies and self-help practices can be helpful in some areas of our lives, they are often not sufficient to help us heal in other areas. Many of us who have experienced emotional trauma have spent a lifetime in therapy, reading books, and trying different strategies in an effort to heal. Although we may have experienced some benefit from them, many of us still struggle. Why?

What I have come to understand is that emotional trauma impacts three different parts of us simultaneously:

1. The emotional circuits in the brain, which causes us to experience dysregulated emotions.
2. The development of our core self-concept, which causes us to have a distorted perception of ourselves.
3. The way that we form emotional attachment bonds with others, which leads to difficulties in relationships.

Unless all three parts are addressed on our healing journey, we will tend to get stuck. For example, eye movement desensitization and reprocessing therapy (EMDR) may help us calm our nervous system so we have fewer flashbacks, but it won't help us develop a healthier self-concept. Therapy to heal our sense of self will have limited benefit in helping us form healthier emotional bonds with our partners. If we are stuck in our trauma in one part of our lives, it tend to will undermine our ability to heal in the others. However, if we address all three of these areas at the same time—emotional dysregulation, a distorted self-concept, and disrupted attachment—we can make huge progress in our healing journey in a relatively short period of time.

The information in this book details what I have come to understand about emotional trauma—both as someone who has personally struggled with its effects and as a licensed therapist who has worked with traumatized clients—particularly in the context of committed relationships. I wish that I could have read this book forty years ago when I was so lost and disoriented. It would have provided me with a framework for understanding my experience and a strategy for moving forward on my path to healing in an intentional way. Although this information was not available when I started my journey, my hope is that what you learn here will save you years of struggle and facilitate your healing.

The Trauma Word

It is common for those of us who have experienced emotional neglect, bullying, abuse, exposure to domestic violence, housing instability, and inadequate or shame-based parenting in childhood to struggle with the idea that we were traumatized. Instead, we tend to see our low self-esteem, trouble setting boundaries, relationship difficulties, depression, or being overly emotional as "just who we are." Seeing ourselves as living with the effects of trauma may take some time. I know it was certainly the case for me, and has been the case for many of my clients.

Many of us struggle to recognize that certain experiences are traumatic because of the way the brain tries to normalize our experience. The human mind is extremely good at adapting to whatever conditions in which it finds itself—even if those conditions are harsh and dehumanizing. Over time, it will tend to accept just about anything as normal. This is especially true in childhood when we have no frame of reference that we can use to evaluate whether our experience is normal or healthy. It often isn't until we go to therapy or begin sharing our experience with others that we realize how earlier experiences may be impacting our life today.

Acknowledging that we have experienced trauma can also be hard because it leads us to reevaluate many things in life, such as "What does this mean about me?," "Does this make me broken?," "What does this mean about my family and my relationship with them?," and "Where does this fit in my sense of who I am?" This reevaluation of how we understand ourselves can be difficult and disorienting as it often involves a deep level of questioning everything we think and feel.

Do You Have Emotional Trauma?

Those of us who have experienced emotional trauma tend to share some common experiences. As you go through this list of questions, I invite you to pay attention to how many of these resonate with you.

Do you often:

1. Feel like you don't belong, even when you are with a group?
2. Experience derealization or feel like you are living in a dream state?
3. Have episodes of lost time or can't remember the past few minutes?

4. Struggle to maintain focus or have been diagnosed with ADHD?
5. Regularly experience nightmares or night terrors?
6. Often feel like you have to guess at what normal is?
7. Have trouble calming yourself down when you become upset?
8. Feel like you are constantly trying to figure out who you are?
9. Struggle with addiction to drugs, sex, alcohol, food, or gambling?
10. Sometimes feel flooded with distress, anger, or fear that is overwhelming?
11. Engage in self-harming behavior, such as cutting?
12. Feel terrified of people or find it difficult to trust?
13. Experience disturbing or intense intrusive thoughts?
14. Emotionally shut down or feel like you want to run away?
15. Have trouble setting boundaries?
16. Experience an ill-defined sense of urgency to be somewhere else?
17. Pick the wrong partners in relationships?
18. Feel like your emotions are always on high alert?
19. Sacrifice your own well-being to prove your worthiness to other people?
20. Struggle with racing thoughts and extreme swings in emotion?
21. Avoid certain people, places, or situations that trigger painful memories?

22. Work toward a goal and then undermine your own success?
23. Struggle to form and maintain intimate relationships?
24. Feel like there is just something about you that is broken and unlovable?
25. Feel like life has no meaning?

If you read through this list and the questions really seemed to resonate, you are probably living with the effects of emotional trauma.

Is Your Experience "Real Trauma"?

There is a natural tendency to minimize the significance of our own experiences when we hear the horrible things that other people have experienced. We may feel that what we went through wasn't as bad as what other people have gone through, so maybe our experience wasn't "real trauma." It's important to understand that emotional trauma is an effect, not an event. In other words, it is not about the severity of what happened, it is about how our nervous system and sense of self was affected by the events. Not everyone will be affected by emotional neglect, violence, or abuse in the same way. Factors such as social support, our genetic makeup, emotional connection with our family, and individual temperament will make some of us more sensitive to trauma while others may be more resilient. There is also considerable evidence that some of the effects of emotional trauma in our parents may be passed down genetically through a process called epigenesis.

Because our brains will try to normalize just about any situation, regardless of how insane or harmful, it may be difficult for us to initially recognize that our family life may have had a detrimental impact on us. The reality is that it doesn't matter whether we think the events in our lives were hurtful enough to qualify as "real trauma." The important thing to focus on is whether you experience the effects of trauma. If you have the symptoms, then your experience qualifies.

Some of the stories in this book are about people who survived pretty extreme events and were deeply impacted by them, but it is important to remember that you don't need a history of extreme violence or abuse to suffer from the effects of trauma. Those who grew up with emotionally uninvolved or absent parents, were moved from home to home in foster care, or were shamed and mocked will often struggle with many of the same emotional and psychological challenges as those whose abuse was more extreme.

Recovering from Emotional Trauma

I would like to start by saying that recovering from emotional trauma is entirely possible. I have done it, many others have done it, and you can do it, too. Healing doesn't happen overnight, and the work to recover can be difficult at times. But, if you are willing to step out of your comfort zone and take certain actions, even if imperfectly, you can release yourself from the effects of emotional trauma and live the life you want. It doesn't mean that you will never get triggered or experience difficult emotions. You will. The difference is that by having the right tools, you will be able to navigate through those experiences in a healthier way.

Your journey of recovery from emotional trauma has three parts: calming your emotions, healing your core self-concept, and strengthening your relationships.

Calming your emotions is achieved by shifting the emotional circuits in your brain out of being stuck in the fight-or-flight response and reduce your levels of anxiety and stress. You will learn how to become more grounded in your body, create a sense of safety and agency, and process through traumatic memories.

Healing your core self-concept focuses on repairing the parts of your sense of self that have been damaged or undeveloped. By learning ways to develop a sense of value, connection, and a clear sense of identity, you will find the feelings of being unlovable, broken, and helpless that are so common with emotional trauma start to disappear. Through a series of exercises, you will learn techniques to identify specific parts of your sense of self that have been affected, and how to heal that part of yourself.

Strengthening our relationships comes through learning new communication skills that help us emotionally attune to other important people in our lives and to navigate through conflict in a healthier way. This relational part of our recovery is very important. Strong and stable emotional attachment bonds to partners, close friends, family members, or therapists play a large role in our ability to heal. The sense of connection calms the alert circuits in the brain, alleviates the sense of loneliness, and helps us heal our sense of self.

How This Book Is Organized

This book is organized into two parts. In first half of the book, we define emotional trauma and how different forms of trauma may impact us differently. We talk about the three dimensions of emotional trauma—emotional dysregulation, damage to our core self-concept, and difficulty with relationships—and how each of these tends to show up in our lives.

In the second half of the book, we discuss how to recover from emotional trauma. I show you how to heal the three dimensions of emotional trauma by calming your nervous system, repairing the damage to your core self-concept, and learning some skills to help you navigate relationships more effectively.

In the last chapter, we will take everything that we learned and create our personal journey of recovery. Everyone has unique experiences, has been affected by emotional trauma in their own way, and needs different things in order to heal. Your journey of recovery will be about clarifying where your wounded parts are, prioritizing where to focus your energy, and creating a plan for healing that is aligned with your needs and goals.

My Hope for You

I wrote this book to help people like you heal from the effects of emotional trauma. This book is about what I learned on my healing journey, both as someone who has lived with the effects of trauma and also as a professional therapist who has helped many people recover from its effects. With this personal and professional background, I not only understand trauma's impact from an academic standpoint, I have also lived it. In the following pages, you will learn what emotional trauma is, how it affects you, and the specific things that you can do to help yourself heal.

I should note that this is not a comprehensive textbook on every available trauma therapy. Most approaches to healing tend to work well in some situations and not as well in others. Just as there is no single tool that can build a house, there is not a single therapy or self-help technique that will heal all forms of trauma. What I present to you here is what I have found helpful in my own healing and with clients who have experienced emotional trauma.

Having lived through the debilitating effects of trauma for much of my life, I appreciate what that experience is like. I have done my best to accurately describe the felt experience of living with dysregulated emotions, a damaged core sense of self, and difficulty with relationships. I also offer the message that you don't have to live with the effects of trauma forever. There is hope.

It is not your fault that you experienced emotional trauma. That was out of your control. What is in your control is what you will do going forward. My hope is that the information in the following pages will help you build a better version of yourself, create relationships that last, and experience the kind of life that you were meant to have. Let's get to work.

CHAPTER 2

What Is Emotional Trauma?

THROUGHOUT HISTORY AND IN every corner of the world, people have recognized that something happens to the human soul when we are exposed to certain types of stress. This seems to be true whether we are physically injured or not. The first written account of the impact of emotional trauma is in the Epic of Gilgamesh, dating back to 2100 BCE. In the story, the main character Gilgamesh witnesses the death of his closest friend, Enkidu. Gilgamesh is so tormented by this event that he experiences recurrent and intrusive thoughts, nightmares, and a sense of dread. His confrontation with death dramatically changed his personality and held his mind prisoner to the horrors he witnessed.

During the Napoleonic Wars in the early 1800s, French physicians described what they called *"vent du boulet"* syndrome (literally "wind of the cannonball"), in which soldiers simply collapsed into a prolonged stupor due to the terrifying sound of cannonballs whizzing past them. Even though the soldiers had no physical injury, they were unable to stand or function and just lay there frozen. The extreme and inescapable distress of war caused their nervous system to become overwhelmed and shut down.

In 1894, William James, considered to be one of the founding fathers of psychology alongside Pierre Janet and Wilhelm Wundt, called experiences of extreme psychological distress "thorns in the spirit." These thorns were not physical wounds, but emotional wounds that could arise from intensely frightening and inescapable events that overwhelmed the brain's ability to cope. James recognized that once these psychological experiences occur, they often create a long-term change in people's mental and emotional lives.

French psychologist Pierre Janet observed that what defined a traumatic experience wasn't the severity of the event, but how our mind was affected by it. In his 1899 book, *L'automatisme Psychologique*, Janet wrote that "the trauma was not the event itself, but the reaction of the individual", meaning that trauma cannot be determined by some external measure of severity, but rather by how the nervous system of the individual responded to the event. Therefore, an event that was traumatic for one person may not be traumatic for another. The trauma experience is unique to each individual. Janet further observed how an individual who has experienced trauma is "unable to integrate the traumatic memories" and that those people "lose their capacity to integrate other experiences." He noted how people who have experienced trauma "seem to have the evolution of their lives halted" as if parts of them are anchored in time and unable to move forward.

In their book *Studies on Hysteria*, German psychologists Josef Breuer and Sigmund Freud described the effects that childhood sexual trauma had on the lives of adult women. Hysteria was a condition in women, primarily in the Germanic countries, where they would faint, be unable to speak, or where parts of their body would become paralyzed for no apparent reason. Fascinated by this, Freud and Breuer asked these women to tell them their stories. Based on what the women told them, they theorized that the symptoms these women experienced were likely due to a severe unconscious stress response to sexual trauma that they had experienced as children. Freud wrote:

> In every analysis of a case of hysteria based on sexual traumas, we find that impressions from the pre-sexual period which produced no effect on the child, attain traumatic power at a later date as memories when the girl or married woman has acquired an understanding of sexual life.

Although the effects of trauma on soldiers had been studied in both world wars, the interest in psychological trauma grew significantly during the Vietnam War as soldiers returned home from the jungles of Southeast Asia. Although many returning soldiers had no physical injuries, many of them suffered debilitating mental and emotional consequences from their experience. Despite political resistance to accepting psychological trauma as a real phenomenon, the term post-traumatic stress disorder (PTSD) was officially recognized as a condition in the 1980s when it was included in the third edition of the Diagnostic and Statistical Manual of Mental Disorders (DSM-III). PTSD was described as a cluster of symptoms that result from exposure to extreme stress events. Symptoms included flashbacks, intrusive thoughts, hypervigilance, avoiding triggering situations, difficulty feeling positive emotions, nightmares, emotional dysregulation and a sense of hopelessness.

Over the decades that followed, our understanding of trauma has evolved to also include the effects of emotional trauma that occur in children who experience years, if not decades, of repeated abuse, shaming, or emotional neglect within a family system. This chronic pattern of childhood neglect and abuse not only resulted in many of the classic trauma effects associated with PTSD, but it also resulted in a disruption in the development of a healthy self-concept. So, not only did kids struggle from dysregulated emotions, but they also struggled with the effects of a damaged internal model of themselves.

The point here is that emotional trauma is not a new concept. Since our ancestors first began recording history on cuneiform tablets, we have known that distressing events can leave imprints on our minds that affect how we experience life.

Defining Emotional Trauma

Emotional trauma is any inescapable and distressing experience that results in long-term changes in how we feel, think, and behave. It can be in the form of acute trauma, which is a short-term extreme event, such as an assault or exposure to violence, or a more chronic type of attachment trauma, which is experienced as an inescapable pattern of distress over a prolonged period of time, particularly during childhood. Although each of these will affect us differently, what both types of trauma share are the elements of inescapability and emotional distress, and the inability of the brain to integrate the distressing memories. In some forms of trauma, this results in fragments of our experiences splitting off from our conscious awareness, and showing up later as images, sensations, emotions, and body responses that we cannot control. In other forms of trauma, the lack of adequate nurturing leads to parts of our self-concept not developing properly. Let's take a closer look at each of these forms of trauma.

Acute Trauma

Acute trauma is a stress response to an atrocious event or series of events that are intensely horrifying and create an inescapable shock to a person that overwhelms their nervous system. These can be experiences like an airplane crash, sexual assault, combat, domestic violence, witnessing a murder, a life-threatening illness, or anything that is terrifying, intense, and inescapable. Because these experiences are too intense to put into words, it is often very difficult to process and encode them into our long-term memory as an experience that happened in the past. Instead, these unprocessed experiences keep parts of our emotional system stuck in a sustained state of alarm, as though we are experiencing the traumatic event in the here and now. When our emotions are trapped in this alarm state, we will tend to experience problems stemming from emotional dysregulation, as well as the physical impacts of an emotional system stuck in a state of chronic stress.

Let's take a look at a couple of examples. The following two stories come from clients of mine who had experienced pretty significant acute trauma during childhood. Their stories illustrate how these kinds of experiences can create a lasting imprint on their mental and emotional lives.

"I Shot My Uncle"

Roger and Kate came to see me to do something about Roger's anger problem. The two of them had been married for just over six years and had met each other at an Alcoholics Anonymous meeting. About two years into their relationship, Kate began to notice Roger becoming more and more aggressive and paranoid. Although he had not been physically violent toward her, she began to fear him and was afraid that at some point, he may become violent.

Roger had been released from prison for a drug conviction a couple of years before he met Kate, and prior to his arrest, he had been a member of a motorcycle club that was involved with a lot of drug dealing and violence. Although he seemed to avoid sharing any details about his involvement in illegal activities, he did share some of the violence he witnessed or experienced before his arrest. As we explored his childhood, the tone of Roger's voice changed from defensiveness to sadness when he described an event that happened when he was ten years old.

His uncle lived in the house next door, and he and his father would often get into fights when they were drunk. Roger said that one night, he remembers his father and uncle yelling at each other and physically fighting. He remembers walking into the living room to see his father trying to push his uncle out of the front door. Roger ran up to his father and helped push his uncle out of the house, and then quickly slammed the door closed.

A few minutes later, Roger heard his uncle kick in the front door and scream "I am going to kill you" at his father. In a panic, Roger quickly ran into his parents' bedroom, grabbed his father's handgun, and rushed back into the living room where he watched his uncle push his father to the floor and pull out a knife. Roger raised the handgun and fired three shots into his uncle, killing him. Although Roger was never charged with any crime, he was intensely traumatized by the entire event. Shortly afterward, his parents divorced, and Roger ran away from home. After several years of living with various friends, he joined a motorcycle club because, as he said, "I found a place where I belonged."

Once out of prison and sober, Roger became very active in training service dogs for veterans, sponsoring recovering addicts, and regularly volunteering to feed people who were homeless. He described his relationship with Kate as the best thing that had ever happened to him. Unfortunately, the trauma he had experienced as both a child and a young adult still impacted him deeply. Despite trying to do the right thing, he suffered from flashbacks, feelings of intense anger that he couldn't control, difficulty trusting people, and never feeling like he could relax. He kept several guns in his house due to a sense of terror that someone would try to break into their house and attack them.

I referred Roger to another therapist to do individual EMDR therapy, and I worked with the two of them as a couple to help them navigate through Roger's trauma together. Within a few months, Roger became a different person. His demeanor changed, and he seemed less defensive and agitated. He said that he felt much calmer and less paranoid, and Kate said that she felt closer to him than she had in a long time and said that "he wasn't as angry all the time."

The Masked Intruder

Tyrie was referred to me several years ago from one of her family members who was concerned that she may try to hurt herself. I could tell from our initial conversation that Tyrie was not enthused about speaking to a therapist and seemed very guarded in her responses. After a couple of sessions, she reluctantly began to share some of her story with me about what it was like for her growing up.

Tyrie grew up in a home where her father was frequently absent and seemed completely disinterested in her. Her mother was very critical, and Tyrie felt like she could never do anything right. Whenever her mother was upset, she would become very emotionally abusive and mean toward Tyrie, often for reasons that Tyrie said "were completely made up in my mom's head." In one of our sessions, Tyrie described an event that was particularly traumatizing.

> When I was about seven or eight years old, my mother told me she was going to the store and that she would be right back. A few minutes after she was gone, my mom put on a mask and pretended to break into our house. I was so scared. Once she got in, she came after me like she was going to kill me. I froze and was lying on the floor screaming and shaking. Then my mom took off her mask and she made fun of me for being so scared.

The intense terror and shock that Tyrie experienced from thinking that an intruder was going to kill her is mind-numbing to think about. The fact that her mother intentionally did this to her and then mocked her for being afraid is shockingly cruel. It is no wonder that Tyrie struggled with depression, panic attacks, feeling unlovable, and engaging in self-harming behaviors. For years, she cut herself, and used drugs and sex to "numb out." She said that the only time she felt like she was worth anything was when, as she said, "men used my body for sex because that's the only thing that I can do right." After a string of failed relationships, she said that she just wasn't interested in having friends anymore and was more comfortable alone.

While the experiences of Roger and Tyrie are pretty intense, the reality is that most people have experienced an acute traumatic event in their life. This may be in the form of a rape, surviving a dog attack, being bullied, or any variety of experiences where you are trapped and terrified.

While it is easy to appreciate how a shocking event can have a devastating effect on someone's mental and emotional life, there is another form of trauma that is often harder to see. This form of trauma occurs within a family system where the critical emotional bond between parent and child is either absent or toxic. This is referred to as attachment trauma.

Attachment Trauma

Attachment trauma is a form of chronic emotional trauma, primarily during childhood, that impacts the development of the person's self-concept and their ability to form and maintain healthy relationships. This can be in the form of aggression or deprivation, and typically results from living with emotional abandonment, shame-based parenting, verbal abuse, role reversal where the child becomes the caregiver for the parent, an unstable or inconsistent home life, or any other disruption in the parent-child attachment bond that leaves a negative impact on a child's self-concept and interferes with their ability to form and maintain healthy attachment relationships. It can also occur when a child's life is so highly structured or controlled by their parents that they do not have the opportunity or encouragement to develop an internalized structure of the self.

WHAT IS EMOTIONAL TRAUMA?

When our core sense of self is not nurtured properly, we will tend to feel a sense of being flawed, unlovable, unworthy, like a mistake, and may experience feelings of isolation and chronic loneliness. We may suffer from a chronic low-level depression that makes life feel colorless, unsatisfying, or meaningless. Many struggle to find a sense of who they are, feel a sense of existential disorientation, engage in people-pleasing behaviors, feel a sense of emotional isolation, and may sometimes feel rudderless and lost.

Unlike acute trauma, where the distress comes from some perceived external danger, the distress from attachment trauma comes from holes in our core self-concept that create a distorted perception of what is within us. In other words, rather than being terrified about something attacking you, there is an internalized sense that you are broken, are unlovable, or that there is something fundamentally wrong with you. Those of us with attachment trauma may present well on the outside, but behind the carefully crafted social presentation, many of us carry a hole in our soul that permeates every corner of our lives. This form of emotional trauma emerges whenever there is inadequate emotional nurturing from our caregivers during childhood, as in the case of emotional neglect, or when our sense of self is actively undermined by our caregivers through mocking and shaming. Let's take a closer look at the two most common forms of attachment trauma: emotional neglect and shame-based parenting.

Emotional Neglect

Emotional neglect typically happens when parents are emotionally or physically absent, or when parents are not emotionally invested in their children's lives. This often happens when:

1. Parents have an active addiction, such as to alcohol, drugs, or gambling.

2. Parents are too preoccupied with their own lives to adequately attend to the emotional lives of their children.
3. Parents are emotionally immature and lack the skills to engage with their kids in a healthy way.
4. Family systems place all of the attention on superficial topics rather than on how children are doing emotionally.
5. Parents are either deceased or struggling with a major illness.
6. Kids live in an unstable environment as in the case of foster care or being shuttled between various family members.
7. Parents attempt to control too much of their child's life.

Emotional neglect often leaves us with a poorly formed sense of self, difficulty identifying our emotions, struggling to emotionally attune to others, a tendency to pick emotionally unavailable partners, and no intuitive sense of how to successfully navigate intimate relationships.

The story of my friend David illustrates one way in which emotional neglect can affect us and our ability to form and maintain relationships.

"I Don't Know How to Pick Women"

David was standing in his kitchen when it hit him that his third marriage was over. He stared blankly down at the pan of sauce cooking on the stove. Expressionless. Silent. Numb. He had invited me over to talk—to make sense out of what happened. His wife had just moved out in an act of contempt in what was the latest chapter of the same old story. A story that always opened with excitement, happiness, and love when he met someone new, but inevitably ended the same way.

"Why do I keep picking fucked-up women?" he asked while staring at the pan. "There is something in me that is attracted to the crazy ones."

David grew up in a wealthy neighborhood as the adopted single child of an older couple. While he had every material thing that he could ever want, the one thing that his parents never gave him was their emotional investment. Like everything else in his parents' lives, David was a possession. He was an object that helped his parents feel good about themselves. While they fed him with a lot of expensive things, they starved him from the warmth, emotional connection, and nurturing that he so desperately wanted.

At the time, David had a Ferrari, a big house, and a massive collection of rare guns, but he was crippled by the damage resulting from the emotional neglect he experienced growing up. He struggled with intense bouts of self-hatred and fits of anger, and he struggled to keep friends. Despite being a very intelligent and generous man, he lacked an innate sense of how to attract a healthy partner or how to successfully navigate through a relationship.

In all three of his failed marriages, the women he ultimately married seemed wonderful at first, but over time the relationships all crumbled. For example, in his first marriage, his wife had numerous affairs, and when David discovered them, she blamed him, as though it was his fault that she cheated on him.

In his second marriage, he filed for divorce one week after the wedding ceremony when his wife had a psychotic break and came after him with a knife. When I asked about that, he said he should have suspected something was wrong when she never allowed him to spend the night until they were married. He joked, "I suppose she couldn't keep up the facade of sanity for more than a few hours at a time."

In his third marriage, his wife constantly belittled him and made him feel like he couldn't do anything right. Her aggression toward him escalated until she moved out one day in a final bitter demonstration of how much of a failure he was as a husband and a human being.

When we sat down to eat, he told me that he was done with relationships.

"Everyone I date ends up being a psycho," he said. "I just don't know how to pick women."

David didn't struggle with the inability to form and maintain intimate relationships because he was a bad guy, or because he was not smart enough, or because he didn't try hard enough. He struggled because the emotional neglect that he experienced during childhood affected his development in a way that made relationships very difficult to navigate. Not only did he pick unhealthy partners, but he lacked an intuitive sense of how to "do relationships." He struggled to communicate, was often emotionally withdrawn, had frequent episodes of explosive anger, and he used alcohol to deal with the distress of his poorly formed sense of self.

Emotional neglect like what Davied experienced is one form of attachment trauma. Let's take a quick look at another form of attachment trauma: shame-based parenting.

Shame-Based Parenting

Shame-based parenting is a style of exercising control over a child that is marked by the use of cutting remarks to make children feel bad about themselves, their worth, or their abilities. This is often through verbal criticism, sarcastic remarks, belittling, or mocking. This kind of toxic shaming from our parents or caregivers often results in us developing an internalized sense that there is something fundamental about us that is flawed, wrong, or unlovable.

It's important to note that toxic shame is not the same as healthy shame. Healthy shame is intended to make us feel bad for something that we have done wrong so that we won't do it again in the future. It is intended to shape our behavior so that we can be more successful in society. When used in this way, healthy shame facilitates social integration and does not damage the sense of self. So, while healthy shame is intended to make you feel bad about what you did wrong, toxic shame makes you feel bad about who you are. Healthy shame helps you be a better person in society, while toxic shame does just the opposite.

Examples of toxic shame include:

1. Being laughed at, mocked, or made to feel stupid.
2. Being belittled or being told that you can't do anything right or are a failure.
3. Feeling like nothing you did is ever good enough.
4. Not being allowed to express emotions or being ridiculed for them.
5. Being blamed for your parents' problems.
6. Being responsible for managing the emotions of your caregivers.
7. Never feeling validated or that your experience was okay.

Those of us who grew up in homes where our parents were shaming and hypercritical will often develop a combination of the feeling of emptiness and worthlessness, coupled with a hair-trigger defensive response toward any perceived attack. We may become defensive or feel like we are being attacked, even when we are not. It is common to feel unsafe opening up to other people, to struggle with trust, or to engage in people-pleasing behavior.

The following story of Becky and Tre is a good example of how this may show up in a relationship.

Flooded with Rage

Becky grew up in a home with an abusive, alcoholic father and an aggressive mother who cycled through periods of depression that would last for weeks, followed by periods of hyperactivity and irritability. Becky was the youngest of three children and the only girl. Although she didn't know all of the details of what happened, there were rumors in the family that shortly after she was born, her mother had an episode of postpartum psychosis. Becky vaguely remembered living with her grandmother for a while when she was very young while her mother was in a hospital, but she didn't remember much else about her early childhood.

Most of her memories from growing up were seeing her mother and older brothers being beat up by her father when he was in a drunken rage, and being threatened by him to "shut up or she would get more of the same" if she cried. Her mother idolized her two brothers and acted like they could never do anything wrong, but would often tell Becky that "she was a mistake" and that she "never wanted to have a girl." Becky said that her mom became increasingly harsh toward her during her teenage years, and during one session she joked, "I think I was grounded for my last two years of high school."

Tre and Becky met during college and immediately hit it off. They grew very close over the next couple of years and decided to get married. Shortly after, they began struggling with conflict that quickly escalated into heated fights. They usually ended when Tre emotionally shut down, Becky became overwhelmed with distress, and the two of them hurled harsh words at each other until one of them walked away. This was usually followed by a couple of days of not talking to each other, and then just going forward as though nothing had happened. Becky finally decided to call to set up an appointment for couple therapy after a particularly heated argument when Tre told her that it was over, left the house, and went to stay at a hotel.

After a few sessions, a pattern in their relationship became clear. Tre would say something that triggered a trauma response in Becky, and Becky would become very aggressive and defensive.

"It's like she becomes a different person," Tre said. "I can see it in her face as soon as it happens, and I just think to myself, 'Oh God, here it comes.'"

Becky described her experience during those times, saying, "I feel a wave of rage flow over me. I can feel it happen, but I can't stop it."

She also struggled with intense feelings of unlovability, worthlessness, and an ill-defined sense of anxiety, which would often come out in arguments as accusing Tre of not loving her and treating her like she didn't matter, or saying she felt like he was always attacking her.

Like David in the previous story, Becky's childhood experience had a substantial impact on how she experienced life as an adult. In both cases, emotional trauma from childhood led to problems in their relationships, their ability to regulate their emotions, and how they felt about themselves.

The bottom line is our experience with our caregivers when we are growing up has a huge impact on our core self-concept and how well we can form and sustain relationships as adults. Our self-concept and relationship patterns will continue to evolve in adulthood, for sure, but healing and growth requires a greater level of intention and effort the older we get.

Acute Trauma vs. Attachment Trauma

Understanding the difference between the symptoms that are associated with acute trauma and attachment trauma will help us better understand our experience and will be helpful in our healing journey. In general, acute trauma tends to have a greater impact on the stress circuits in the brain, whereas attachment trauma tends to impact on our internal self-concept. Let's take a closer look at how each of these tends to affect us differently.

- Acute trauma damages us through inescapable events of extreme stress, whereas attachment trauma damages us through emotional neglect, shame-based parenting, and disrupted attachment.

- Acute trauma has a greater impact on our sense of safety and agency, whereas attachment trauma has a greater impact on our sense of lovability, connection with others, and our sense of identity.

- Acute trauma primarily impacts the alarm circuits in the brain, whereas attachment trauma primarily impacts our self-concept and how we perceive ourselves in relation to the rest of the world.

- Acute trauma tends to be more associated with chronic stress, hypervigilance, nightmares, dysregulated emotions, and avoiding triggering situations, whereas attachment trauma tends to be more associated with internalized shame, relationship difficulties, and the feeling of being a broken or unlovable person.

- Acute trauma can occur at any point when we experience an inescapable and horrifying event, whereas attachment trauma typically happens during childhood experiences with caregivers and peers. However, it can also occur in adulthood when people are stuck in a toxic relationship.

- Acute trauma typically is caused by a single event or events that occur during a confined period of time, whereas attachment trauma tends to occur from a consistent pattern of interaction over a period of many years—particularly during childhood.

- Acute trauma triggers emotional responses from perceived external threats, whereas attachment trauma triggers emotional responses from perceived internal flaws.

How Does Trauma affect you?

Emotional trauma affects us in three fundamental ways. First, trauma causes the emotional circuits of the brain to become stuck in a state of high alert. This is due to the way memories of trauma are stored in the brain. Trauma memories are not processed the same way that normal memories are processed. Instead of being encoded in our memory as a coherent story of something that happened in the past, the emotions, smells, sounds, and sensations of the event become dissociated from our conscious awareness and are reexperienced as disorganized fragments of sensations that cause the body to react as though the trauma was happening in the here and now. This is the emotional dysregulation part of trauma.

Second, it impacts the structure of our core self-concept. This internal structure can be thought of as a set of psychological boundaries that we create as a way of organizing our experiences, how we make sense of the world, and how we shape our self-perception. Boundaries are the emotional and mental limits we set to define our sense of self and protect our well-being. They help us to differentiate ourselves and to establish the edge between where we end and another person begins. Each of us has two sets of boundaries that we develop throughout our lifetime: external boundaries and internal boundaries.

External Boundaries

External boundaries are the limits we set with our partners in relationships and with other people in society. These boundaries define our interpersonal distance from others, how we perceive ourselves in relationship to the world around us, how much we are willing to give or receive, and what we will or will not tolerate. Whereas our internal boundaries are the rules that organize our internal world, our external boundaries are the rules that organize our external world. External boundaries are developed through modeling from our parents and peers while growing up, and they are critical for protecting our emotional, mental, physical, and material well-being. They are intended to help us:

- Manage our personal space and privacy.
- Interpret our relationship to the world around us.
- Set limits on how much emotional work we are willing to invest in a relationship.
- Respect differences of opinion without feeling personally attacked.
- Say "no" when we are already overcommitted or need time for ourselves.
- Communicate our sexual desires, needs, and limits with our partner.
- Set limits on lending money or sharing possessions with others.
- Decide not to engage in gossip or interpersonal drama.

Acute trauma is an event that violates our external boundaries. It bowls over our ability to maintain our personal space and violates our personal integrity. This happens during an assault, childhood abuse, exposure to violence, major accidents, being bullied, or even a life-threatening illness—any terrifying and inescapable experience that invades our personal space.

Whereas acute trauma acts like a wrecking ball that punches a hole in our external boundaries, attachment trauma often impedes our ability to form healthy external boundaries in the first place.

If we grew up in a home where our environment was unstable, unpredictable, or hostile, or where our parents were emotionally absent, then the intuitive sense of how to set and hold external boundaries may have never fully developed. This is why many of us with attachment trauma struggle with feeling like people take advantage of us, feel disrespected, experience burnout, have difficulty communicating our needs in relationships, tend to be overly-influenced by what other people think, and may give away our resources to our own detriment.

Internal Boundaries

Internal boundaries are the internal framework that helps us regulate and manage our internal experiences so we can maintain a healthy balance between our thoughts, feelings, and behaviors. Unlike external boundaries, which define how we interact with others, internal boundaries are more about self-regulation and personal control. When we have healthy internal boundaries, we have the ability to:

- Self-regulate our emotions, which allows us to manage emotion without being overwhelmed.
- Avoid doing things that may sabotage our own success, like procrastination or engaging in unhealthy habits.
- Resist impulsive behavior, allowing us to pause and reflect before acting.
- Maintain focus and resist being derailed by distraction.
- Give ourselves permission to make mistakes without spiraling into guilt or shame.
- Stay true to our values and beliefs, even in difficult situations.

- Establish and follow rules for ourselves in things like time management, diet, and personal growth.

When we experience attachment trauma, our internal structure of the self often does not form in a healthy way, if at all. For this reason, many people will find it difficult to self-regulate emotion, tend to do things that ultimately sabotage their own success, act impulsively, experience a lot of guilt and self-shame, violate their own ethics, and have difficulty organizing their time and maintaining discipline.

Emotional trauma damages this internal framework of the self—the complex of internal and external boundaries that defines who we are and how we manage our place in the world. Although acute trauma, such as an assault, will damage our internal framework differently than the chronic trauma, both types of emotional trauma are harmful specifically because of the way they violate or damage our internal and external boundaries. When external boundaries are violated or don't form properly, our brain tends to get stuck in a fight-or-flight response. When internal boundaries are violated or don't form properly, we tend to struggle with a sense of loneliness, disconnection, and worthlessness.

The third way trauma affects us is that it impacts how we are able to form and sustain attachment relationships. Difficulty in creating and maintaining attachment bonds often starts early in childhood when our emotional attachment to our parents is disrupted in some way, or we experience attachment trauma. Disrupted childhood attachment bonds not only impacts the emotional system in our brain and the core self, but also impacts the way in which we form attachment bonds in adulthood. We will discuss this in much greater detail in the Difficulty with Relationships chapter.

Abusive or Dysfunctional Families

Acute trauma and attachment trauma happens simultaneously in many families. This is because poor emotional attunement between parents, and between parents and children, is often associated with elevated levels of conflict, violence, instability, or abuse. The combination of the two is particularly damaging because those who we turn to for support and comfort become the source of pain and distress. At the same time, the emotional connection with our parents that we need to help us develop our sense of self and our ability to self-regulate is absent. Therefore, not only are we trapped in a family system that is emotionally or physically unsafe, but the emotional resources that we need to help us develop are absent.

Kids who grow up in this kind of environment often struggle with a very disorganized relationship style and may experience extreme and unpredictable mood swings. The impact this has on us will depend on the severity of the abuse, how often it occurs, how old we are when it happens, our relationship to the abuser, and whether we have any access to support. Typically, exposure that is more frequent, more severe, committed by people who are closer to us, and at a younger age will all tend to affect us more profoundly.

The following story is about a client I had several years ago who had experienced significant acute and attachment trauma during her childhood.

"I Feel So Broken Inside"

Marilyn had been an inmate in the federal prison system for almost ten years when she first contacted me. Her heart-wrenching story of extreme childhood trauma and abusive relationships was nothing short of tragic. One of the exercises I had her do was to write about her childhood and how she thought it affected her. Here is a segment from what she wrote:

> While most kids had parents who read to them, mine thought it was funny to blow pot smoke in my face. While most had family and friends who helped them celebrate their birthdays, my father's friend raped me. While most had sleepovers with other neighborhood kids, my sleepover consisted of my mom and me hiding at her friend's house terrified for our lives, while her friend's oldest son molested me at night. While most kids learned to fish, ride bikes, or camp, my father taught me how to use drugs with him so he wouldn't have to use them alone. So, is this why I have struggled with not knowing who I am, and not knowing how to make good decisions? Is this why I ended up being involved with abusive men whose psychosis felt oddly comfortable and familiar? Or even why I ended up using drugs?
>
> I certainly did not enter either of my abusive relationships because I liked having a tooth busted out with a butt of a gun, or because I liked being choked to unconsciousness and raped, or that I liked being held hostage by a "family friend" in a hotel room for days at a time while being tortured. I ended up in these situations because these sick people had an energy about them that felt familiar, and I felt attracted to them in some way.
>
> In one of my attempts to escape, my abusive ex-boyfriend drove me off the road and fired several shots into my car in an attempt to kill me. And despite my repeated attempts to get away, he always found me. One night, someone hijacked my car when I was stopped at a light, drove me to a cemetery, made me kneel down on the grass, and put a gun to my head. I fully surrendered myself to the realization that I was going to die that night. The only reason why I am alive to write this today is because his gun jammed. Is all of this why I can't think straight, or why I struggle to trust people?
>
> What I want more than anything is a chance for a normal life. I just feel so broken inside. I don't know what to do.

WHAT IS EMOTIONAL TRAUMA?

There are many traumatic experiences that cause both acute trauma and attachment trauma, particularly when a traumatic event occurs within a relational context. The experience of sexual assault is one example where both the nervous system and the sense of self is often damaged. For many, this may result in rape trauma syndrome, which includes the flashbacks and emotional dysregulation of acute trauma, but also the internalized shame, anger, and sense of worthlessness of attachment trauma. There is a condition called complex PTSD that results from repetitive, inescapable trauma that also has characteristics of both PTSD and attachment trauma. These include experiences of human trafficking, slavery, torture, genocide campaigns, or chronic domestic violence. A common factor that is shared by all types of emotional trauma is the sense of helplessness and being trapped.

Key Points to Remember

The most important idea to remember is that trauma happens to normal and healthy brains that are trapped in unhealthy or dangerous situations. When this happens, there are times when the emotional reactions from our trauma can take over and push us out of the driver's seat of our own lives. The ultimate goal is to learn how we can stay in the driver's seat so that we can grow into the people we want to be. Having a clear understanding of what trauma is and how it shows up in our lives is an important first step.

Trauma is caused by inescapable experiences that affect us in three ways:

1. Our emotions become dysregulated. The emotional dysregulation effect is the result of the emotional circuits in the brain getting stuck in a state of hyper activation due to experiencing an inescapable shock, as in the case of acute trauma, or a lack of healthy emotional attunement with

our caregivers, as in the case of neglect or shame-based parenting.

2. Our core sense of self can become distorted or may not develop correctly. The damage to our sense of self is the result of some of our core emotional needs not being met, which impacts the way in which our self-concept forms and how we perceive the world around us.

3. Our ability to form and maintain an intimate attachment bond with a loved one becomes disrupted. The impact on our ability to form and maintain healthy intimate relationships in adulthood is the result of the lack of stable and secure attachment bonds with our caregivers.

Each of these effects contributes to an overall constellation of challenges that can show up in our lives in many different ways, depending on our personality, the severity of our emotional trauma, and access to other support systems growing up.

Over the next three chapters, we will explore the three parts of our lives that are impacted by the effects of emotional trauma:

- Dysregulated emotions
- Damage to our core self-concept
- Disruption in how we form attachment relationships

The goal is to give us a good understanding about how trauma shows up in our lives to help us in our overall journey of recovery.

CHAPTER 3

Our Dysregulated Emotions

THOSE OF US WITH emotional trauma usually have a difficult time with emotions—experiencing them, controlling them, and for many, just being able to identify or label them accurately. We may suffer from persistent sadness, explosive or unexpressed anger, suicidal thoughts, or becoming flooded with distress. We may go emotionally numb, experience sexual inhibition or compulsion, have uncontrollable episodes of crying, and lack an intuitive sense of how to appropriately react in certain circumstances. We may be unable to manage sudden changes in our emotions, struggle to calm down after emotional highs or lows, or struggle to feel any sense of happiness or joy. We may struggle with road rage, maintaining focus, impulsive spending, rapidly shifting from feelings of excitement and joy to a feeling of emotional collapse, or have sudden outbursts of defensiveness that seem disproportionate or oddly out of context.

We experience these things because a traumatized brain processes emotion differently than a nontraumatized one. Trauma convinces us that we are in danger when we are actually safe and distorts our perception of ourselves and the world around us. Unprocessed trauma memories may be triggered at any time and flood us with intense and distressing emotion. This has major consequences when it comes to how we experience our lives, the state of our mental health, and our ability to function in relationships. Before getting into how trauma affects the emotional circuits in the brain, it will be helpful to define what emotions are and why we have them in the first place.

What Is an Emotion?

Emotions are complex states of experience that arise from the limbic system in the brain and are intended to organize our physical and psychological experience into a felt sense of being alive. They provide meaning to everyday life and influence how we adapt to the world in which we live. They saturate every aspect of our existence throughout our lifetime and can either be the engine behind the realization of our potential, or serve as an obstacle to our success. Emotions lie at the core of how we navigate our relationships with others, shape the development of our self-concept, and define our quality of life.

Our relationship with our emotions begins the moment we enter this world and is shaped by our interaction with our parents and environment. As young children, we rely on our parents and caregivers to act like an emotional mirror to help us make sense of our experience and how we should respond. Parents who can emotionally attune to us will help calm our limbic system and help us develop an intuitive sense of what we are feeling. I saw an example of this emotional mirroring while I was having a cup of coffee outside a café.

The Tripping Toddler

I was sitting outside of one of the neighborhood cafés many years ago when I saw a toddler stomping his way up the sidewalk as fast as his little legs could go. He had a look of excitement on his face like he just discovered that he could run, and was like, *Hey! Wow! Check this out! Look at what I can do!* His mom was casually walking a few steps behind him. At one point, I saw the toddler trip on an uneven spot on the sidewalk and fall forward onto his little outstretched hands. He looked shocked, like he was thinking, *What the hell was that?*

With a confused look on his face, he turned back to look at his mother. His mother, seeing him tumble forward, hurried over to him and with a big smile on her face assured him that he was okay. She picked him up off the ground, stood him up in front of her, brushed the dust off his hands, and comforted him. The toddler stared at his mother's face for a few seconds, calmed down, and then started to smile. In less than a minute, the whole interaction was over, and the youngster was happily stomping down the sidewalk once again.

His look of confusion when he hit the ground suggested that his developing brain was trying to figure out how to interpret what had happened. Is this a bad thing? Am I hurt? Should I be scared? By his mother remaining calm and smiling at him, she communicated to her little son that he was okay and that he didn't need to be afraid. This calmed the emotional circuits in his brain. He then encoded a critical emotional memory of the event that would impact the way he experienced events well into the future.

Now imagine the same scenario, but this time, instead of the mother being responsive and comforting, she ignored the fact that he fell and just walked past him, and left him to deal with the experience on his own. What if she freaked out and rushed to her son with a look of terror on her face that he was hurt, or angrily grabbed him by the arm and hit him? How would each of these different responses have affected the toddler's emotional experience of falling down?

The point here is that the ways in which our parents and caregivers interacted with us in childhood will have a significant impact on how we develop the ability to self-regulate as adults. When parents are emotionally dysregulated, emotionally absent, or rage at their child, the child will tend to become very distressed and dissociate from their emotions. If this happens often enough, the child will grow into an adult who has difficulty regulating or even experiencing their emotions. Emotional trauma, particularly in the form of acute trauma, primarily affects a part of our central nervous system called the autonomic nervous system.

The Autonomic Nervous System

The autonomic nervous system is the part of your brain that is responsible for managing all of the systems in your body that keep you alive, such as your blood pressure, heart rate, sleep cycle, breathing, and stress response. In other words, all of the stuff that the brain does that we don't have to think about. The brain does these things automatically, hence the name autonomic nervous system.

The autonomic nervous system is divided into two parts that are normally in balance with each other: the parasympathetic nervous system and the sympathetic nervous system. Understanding these two divisions of your nervous system will give you some insight into how your history of trauma may be impacting your brain and body today, and will help explain why certain healing strategies seem to work while others don't.

A way to think about what these two parts of your nervous system do is to consider the tasks you face in everyday life. There are times when your body needs to be activated to confront the world (work, avoid danger, exercise, and deal with difficulty) and times when your body needs to relax (eat, sleep, have sex, learn, heal, and engage with friends). Each of these states of activation and relaxation are handled by the different parts of our autonomic nervous system.

The Parasympathetic Nervous System

The parasympathetic nervous system can be thought of as the calming system or "rest and digest" system in the brain. It is the division of your nervous system that organizes your mental, emotional, and physical state during times of relaxation, comfort, and healing. The parasympathetic nervous system is the dominant system when we eat, sleep, learn, engage with loved ones, take a walk in the woods, have sex, read, engage in hobbies, and do the things that we normally associate with "feeding our soul." While the sympathetic nervous system gets you ready for battle, the parasympathetic nervous system helps you heal.

The Sympathetic Nervous System

The sympathetic nervous system can be thought of as the "alert system." It organizes our mental, emotional, and physical state in a way that helps us deal with the special challenges of confronting a world that is often chaotic, unpredictable, and dangerous. In situations where we feel threatened, anxious, or afraid, our sympathetic nervous system activates an alarm response—also known as the "fight, flight, freeze, or fawn response." This emotional response triggers an automatic series of actions to help us survive a life-threatening event, such as an assault, animal attack, accident, or any situation where we perceive ourselves to be in danger. It also can be triggered when we experience some perceived threat to our emotional connection with our loved ones. Whenever we perceive a threat, either physically or emotionally, the alarm response may become activated and directs how we think, feel, and act.

Let's take a quick look at each of the four dimensions of the alarm response: fight, flight, freeze, and fawn.

The Fight Response

With the fight response, we are trying to cope with a perceived threat to our wellbeing through confrontation. We usually feel a sense of anger or rage emerge from our gut, and we will try to deal with the threat through verbal confrontation or physical violence. The fight response can get triggered when we don't feel heard, we are disrespected, or our relationship feels in jeopardy.

The Flight Response

With the flight response, we are attempting to cope with a perceived threat to our wellbeing by separating ourselves from the threat. When the flight response takes over, we may feel ourselves emotionally shut down to avoid conflict, and we may physically remove ourselves from the situation. It is also what keeps us from having difficult conversations and advocating for ourselves.

The Freeze Response

With the freeze response, we are attempting to cope with a perceived threat by dissociating from the situation. This can feel like our brain going offline or becoming so overwhelmed with distress that we can't intentionally think, speak, or act. It is as though our insides just turn into a buzzing cloud of static.

The Fawn Response

With the fawn response, we are trying to cope with a perceived threat from someone by appeasing them. This typically occurs in abusive relationships or when we are being held in captivity, where we try to befriend an abuser or threatening individual in order to avoid them becoming upset with us and attacking us. This has also been described as "trauma bonding" or Stockholm syndrome where we may develop an emotional attachment to an unsafe person as a survival strategy.

Getting Stuck in Sympathetic Dominance

In a typical day with a nontraumatized brain, the sympathetic and parasympathetic nervous systems are active in varying proportion, depending on the circumstance. If we have to have a difficult conversation with a coworker, are stuck in traffic, or are running late, our sympathetic nervous system will be more dominant to help us cope in those stressful situations. But once work is done and we can finally relax a bit and spend some time with our loved ones, our parasympathetic nervous system becomes more dominant as we engage in the things we enjoy.

When we experience emotional trauma, we can become stuck in sympathetic dominance. This means that our limbic system becomes stuck in the alarm response. Many of the symptoms of emotional trauma, such as difficulty relaxing, disrupted sleep, flashbacks, hypervigilance, emotional reactivity, a lack of a sense of joy, digestive problems, and feeling chronically stressed, are all the effects of being stuck in the alarm response.

This happens when unprocessed traumatic memories become triggered and reexperienced as though they are happening in the present. In other words, our brain reacts as though it is in danger, even when it is not. Brain scans have shown that when people experience a traumatic memory, parts of the brain that allow us to differentiate what happened in the past from what is happening in the present go offline, as do the brain areas that allow us to integrate all of the sights, sounds, and other sensations of a traumatic event into a coherent story about what happened. Because of this, traumatic memories are often experiences as disjointed fragments of sensations, smells, sounds, and emotions. Sometimes the only thing that is reexperienced is the emotional distress, which can randomly show up as a diffuse feeling of dread, panic, urgency, or helplessness.

When we are stuck in sympathetic dominance, we will feel in a constant state of alarm and tension. Because the parasympathetic system can't do its job during sympathetic dominance, we may experience a number of symptoms, including disruptions in our sleep, elevated blood pressure, digestive changes, difficulty concentrating, migraines, sexual dysfunction, becoming easily upset, and intense and dysregulated emotions.

Because of the constant release of stress hormones, those stuck in sympathetic dominance can develop heart disease, diabetes, fibromyalgia, or other chronic disease, and unfortunately will usually die early. The reason many traumatized people tend to excessively eat and sleep during times of distress is an unconscious attempt to engage the parasympathetic nervous system to restore some balance. Compulsive or addictive behaviors are often symptoms of unresolved trauma rather than a weakness of character. These are often behaviors that are more driven by a stressed brain trying to calm itself down than by some kind of sickness of the soul.

Let's look at some common ways that emotional trauma can show up in everyday life.

Emotional Flashbacks

With a normal event, the details are encoded into our long-term memory, and we have a sense that the experience happened in the past. When we recall normal memories, we may recall feeling happy or sad and will tend to recall details of the event that were particularly meaningful, but we don't feel like they are currently happening. With trauma, the memories are not encoded properly, so all of the emotions continue to be experienced in the here and now. When trauma memories get triggered, the smells, sensations, sights, and emotions of the traumatic event are pulled into the present and are experienced as though they are happening in the here and now. This is referred to as a flashback and is not something that we can control.

For example, one of my clients who had previously served in the Iraq War talked about how he would feel his body react whenever he heard a popping noise. Even something as simple as hearing an acorn drop onto his tent or hearing a stick fall out of a tree and hit the ground while he was camping would cause him to feel a tightness in his gut and an adrenaline rush. Even though his experience in the Iraq War was many years in the past, the trauma he experienced kept his emotional system reacting as though he were still in an active combat zone. While he knew that he wasn't actually back in Iraq, his emotions responded as though he were. This is an emotional flashback.

A couple who I worked with a few years ago provides another example of how an emotional flashback can show up in everyday life.

"A Fourteen-Year-Old Idiot"

Mark and Kelly came to see me for a problem involving their fourteen-year-old son. The son had been suspended from school for what was typical dumb adolescent behavior. After a few minutes of digging into the details about what happened at school, I didn't have any concern that their son was headed for trouble. His father, Mark, also was not particularly concerned and thought that his son "just acted like a fourteen-year-old idiot."

The conflict started when Kelly and Mark arrived home after picking up their son for being suspended. Mark muttered "What an idiot" as they walked through the front door, and Kelly freaked out. His benign comment triggered something in her that was so distressing that she called me for help.

As they sat in my office, her anger seemed oddly extreme. "I didn't even call him an idiot when he could hear me," Mark said.

So, it wasn't as though Mark had called their son an idiot to his face, and he was not even angry, just disappointed. As I watched her confront him for "shaming and belittling their son," something seemed off. I carefully observed her as she confronted him, and I noticed that her skin was changing. It started to become blotchy and her neck was turning red. It was clear that something was happening to her that ran deeper than what Mark had said about their son.

At one point, I stopped her from continuing and asked what had happened to her. She looked at me bewildered. I told her that it seemed like something deeper was going on and asked her if she had been abused. After an awkward moment of her intensely staring at me, she began to cry and recounted being molested by her grandfather when she was young. She had been living alone with that trauma for decades. When Kelly tried to bring it up with other family members while it was happening, she was shut down and told that she was lying.

Now things made sense. Something about the situation with their son and Mark's comment triggered an unprocessed trauma memory, and her body was responding as though the trauma was happening in the present. That was why she had such a strong response for what seemed to be a relatively benign comment from Mark. It was not her fault. It's not like she had the choice to respond this way or even had any understanding of what was happening. The combination of the stress of her son's suspension and the timing of Mark's comment triggered a trauma response. There simply would have been no way to find a resolution to their conflict without addressing the emotional flooding she was experiencing due to her emotional trauma. I put her in touch with a female trauma therapist so she could begin her healing, and we took a break from couple therapy.

Kelly's experience is not uncommon. When emotional trauma punches holes in our sense of self and dysregulates our emotional system, our trauma memories can become triggered by minor events and we may react in the present as though we are reliving a previous trauma. Sometimes these flashbacks can be so vivid that we actually feel as if the past was transported into the present. Someone who was raped, for example, may have a flashback triggered by the tone of another person's voice, or a particular odor, and suddenly feel like the assault is happening all over again. It may feel like the perpetrator is physically present, and it can suddenly become difficult to connect with reality.

Once this flooding happens, there is often little to do except to try to navigate through the emotions the best we can until the emotional system runs its course. While in a flooded state, we may say or do things that are odd or out of character with how we normally think, feel, and act.

Sudden Uncontrolled Anger

All of us have had times when we were frustrated or angry over some event or comment. In most cases, anger is a response to feeling hurt, dismissed, or threatened in some way. For someone who has not experienced trauma, they can become angry and still retain some control over themselves. When we have been traumatized, however, anger is often experienced as a sudden and overwhelming rage where we can say and do things that are inconsistent with who we normally are. When we become triggered, our trauma response pushes us out of the driver's seat and takes over our thoughts, feelings, and actions. After the trauma response has run its course, and we return to our normal selves, we may feel embarrassed and confused about the way we acted.

An example of this kind of anger outburst happened many years ago when I was a waiter at an upscale restaurant.

"The Wrong Fondue"

A nicely dressed couple was seated in my section, and I could tell by their flirty body language that they were on a date. Their appearance and behavior gave the impression that they were both professionals of some kind and were each fairly well off financially. I approached the table and asked them for their drink order and whether they would like an appetizer. They looked at me with big smiles on their faces and ordered some white wine and a Swiss fondue. I dropped off their drinks and appetizer at their table a few minutes later, then went to check on another table before heading back to the kitchen.

When I came back out into the dining room, the man who had ordered the fondue was trying to catch my attention. I walked over to the table and he politely said that I had brought them a cheddar fondue instead of a Swiss fondue. I apologized for my mistake and said that I would take care of it immediately. I rushed back to the kitchen and in less than five minutes was on my way to their table with a Swiss fondue.

As I approached the table, I saw the man sitting there looking at his date with a shocked look on his face as she was grabbing handfuls of bread from the cheddar fondue and angrily throwing them down onto the table like a toddler in a temper tantrum. She stopped and looked away from me when I reached the table. I exchanged their appetizers and quickly cleaned up the mess. The guy looked at me and said "thank you" in a courteous but concerned tone, and I said that I would be back in a moment to take their order. But, when I came back to the table a few minutes later, the man was gone and the woman was sitting at the table with her head in her hands sobbing. She didn't look up when I paused at the table, so I just left her alone. After about twenty minutes of sitting by herself and crying, she left.

Although this happened decades ago, I still think about it. The woman clearly was having a huge trauma reaction. Her behavior when she was grabbing handfuls of bread and throwing them down on the table was more developmentally typical of a five-year-old in the throes of a temper tantrum than a thirty-year-old professional woman on a date. Because of the way she reacted, I would be willing to bet that something traumatic happened to her when she was young that she carried with her into adulthood, and it continued to impact her life. Despite being a young and beautiful professional woman, it appeared that her success in love was thwarted by trauma reactions that she didn't understand and couldn't control.

Paranoia and Hypervigilance

When our brain is stuck in the fight-or-flight response, we become very attuned to perceived threats. Because of this, we will have a tendency to see threats where none actually exist. For example, we may perceive benign comments from people as insults, feel that the world has singled us out in some way, and feel like nobody cares, people are mean, and the world is generally a hostile place. In relationships, one partner may constantly feel attacked by the other, or that the other partner is doing something to intentionally hurt them. They may also struggle with a deep fear that their partner is having an affair or that they have the intention of leaving them. Because of this, people with a history of emotional trauma may become overly defensive and confrontational or may emotionally shut down and isolate themselves. They often have difficulty trusting anyone and may chronically feel like a victim.

"Her Outburst Came out of Nowhere"

Susan was a slender and fit woman in her thirties, who was casually dressed in jeans, a flannel shirt, and a Nike vest. She came to see me one day for a situation that had happened three days earlier with her wife, Kathy. I introduced myself and asked what brought her in to see me. She leaned forward and with a look of grave concern on her face began to tell me what had happened a couple of nights before. Susan said that it was around midnight and she had been lying in bed trying to get some sleep, but her mind started racing so fast and hard that all she could do was just lie there and stare at the ceiling. As her mind churned, she suddenly became convinced that Kathy was cheating on her.

"All of a sudden, it was like everything clicked," Susan said, "and everything that Kathy had done over the past few days made it obvious to me that she was cheating. It was like everything made sense." Susan laid out the evidence that her racing mind interpreted as some kind of proof that Kathy was cheating. "A couple of days ago," Susan said, "Kathy seemed to be in a hurry to get me out the door," which in Susan's racing mind meant that "Kathy must have had a man in their home that she was trying to hide." Susan went on to describe how a couple of days earlier, "Kathy took a phone call and walked out of the room to talk." Susan said that in her mental state, that could only mean that Kathy must have been having a conversation with another lover and was trying to hide it from her. That night, everything Kathy had done was interpreted by Susan as evidence that her partner was having an affair.

Susan's distress escalated to the point where she leapt out of bed, turned on the light, and aggressively accused Kathy of cheating. Kathy was jolted awake and immediately became terrified. "Her outburst seemed to come out of nowhere," Kathy said, and "she looked like she wanted to hurt me." Things continued to escalate from there. At one point, Susan grabbed a knife and pointed it at Kathy. Then Susan burst into their sleeping son's room and screamed at him that Kathy was a cheater and liar. Kathy eventually got Susan out of their son's room and barricaded herself in the bedroom with their son. Terrified, Kathy called the police for help.

When the police arrived, they recognized Susan as a former officer from their department. She was mortified and deeply embarrassed. Once her emotions calmed down, Susan was shocked by what had happened. "It was like I couldn't tell what was real," she said. "It was like something had taken over my mind and I couldn't control it. I could see myself yelling and freaking out, but in a way, it didn't feel like me."

The intense emotional flooding that Susan experienced and the terror she felt of being abandoned by her partner were the consequence of her experiences growing up, coupled with some traumatic experiences as a police officer. Her parents divorced when she was twelve years old, and her father blamed her mother's mental illness for the reason why he left. Susan's mother suffered from intense anxiety and depression, which Susan described as her mother cycling through periods of being very critical of Susan and then completely emotionally withdrawing.

Her work on the police force also exposed her to a number of situations that were very troubling. In one instance, Susan described being called to a house with other officers to find a bloody scene where a woman's boyfriend had killed her two children. Susan described "feeling changed" after that horrifying situation and often had intrusive images about that scene flash into her mind.

Earlier Trauma Being Pulled into the Present

Emotional trauma can show up as being immersed in feelings or behavior that are from an earlier period in life when a trauma occurred. Trauma during development can keep a part of ourselves stuck in an earlier developmental stage of life, even if the other parts of us continue to develop normally. When those trauma memories are triggered, the feelings and sensations that we had when we were younger get pulled into the present and affect how we act.

I see this all the time in couples who are having an argument in session. It is not uncommon for two educated middle-age professionals to suddenly start acting like combative twelve-year-old kids when they become triggered. When I see this happen, I use this as an opportunity to explore their personal trauma histories and how unprocessed trauma memories may be showing up in the therapy session. When the partners are open to exploring their own histories, we often find that some kind of reaction from earlier neglect, divorce, abuse, or shaming is being pulled into their current pattern of conflict. This is not always the case during a conflict between partners, but it is fairly common.

In some cases with people who have experienced childhood trauma, they may feel like they are actually reverting to an earlier stage in life. This is more common with childhood sexual abuse.

"Going into Little Space"

A few years ago, I had a client named Carrie who was suffering from a profound sense of helplessness, depression, nightmares, and severe anxiety. She was in her mid twenties and, after a failed series of relationships, was living in the basement of her grandmother's house. As we started exploring her history, I noticed that she started talking like a little child. Her voice became higher pitched, she spoke in simpler sentences, and she seemed meek and shy. As we dug deeper into her past, she began to go more into what she called her "little space," which was her childlike persona that emerged when her trauma memories were triggered. During therapy, she talked about how she often emotionally felt like she was a little girl and would sometimes wear a diaper and masturbate to a fantasy of being molested by old men. Over a period of several sessions, it became clear that she had been repeatedly sexually molested by an older family member when she was very young. Although she couldn't articulate a coherent story about what happened, the flashes of memory she could recall, coupled with her behavior and the content of her fantasies, painted a vague picture of the horrors she had been through.

As an adult, Carrie described how she went through a series of emotionally abusive relationships, had difficulty keeping jobs, and felt broken, worthless, and hopeless. She felt attracted to unhealthy men, struggled to set boundaries for herself, suffered from frequent panic attacks, and would isolate herself and withdraw into her little space whenever she started feeling overwhelmed.

In Carrie's case, there were three things that were keeping her stuck: her unprocessed trauma memories, her lack of a sense of safety, and her lack of a sense of agency. I referred her to another therapist for EMDR therapy to help her reprocess her early experiences with abuse, and we worked on helping her create a sense of safety and agency in her life. Within a couple of months, she was no longer going into little space during our sessions, and she started feeling a new sense of confidence.

Emotional Numbing

Emotional numbing is common in those of us who have experienced emotional trauma. The loss of the ability to feel is a way that our brain tries to protect itself from a chronic and overwhelming levels of distress. For most, the experience is like feeling "flat" or emotionally detached, feeling empty and like nothing really matters. We may feel a sense of indifference or apathy for things that should bring us joy, and may just feel like everything in our life is devoid of color and meaning. This is different from depression where we feel intense sadness. With emotional numbing, it's like we feel nothing. It's like our soul has been erased, and we feel may disconnected, indifferent, and distant. Behind the veneer of emotional emptiness is often a seething cauldron of anger, guilt, outrage, fear, horror, and grief that defy language. They are experiences for which there simply are no words. So, we sit alone with our distress and numb out.

"I Just Go Numb"

Barb and Rick came in to see me a few years ago so they could, as they said, "learn how to communicate better." They had been together for less than two years and were hoping to "resolve some issues" before they got married. Rick stated that arguments seemed to come out of nowhere and once they started, they escalated quickly into full-blown fights. He also shared his frustration with their lack of a sex life. He said that she "never seems to want to have sex" and that she just shuts down whenever he brings it up. Barb said that Rick, oftentimes, wouldn't follow through on what he said he would do. Whenever she tried to bring it up, he became defensive and she felt herself become flooded with rage.

We eventually turned to the topic of their sex life, and I asked Barb about her thoughts on that. As soon as I brought that up, I could see something in her change. She seemed to become tense and speak in a more matter-of-fact tone than before. Barb said:

> Sometimes, when he touches me, it's like my body goes numb. I don't want it to because there is a part of me that really wants to have sex, but my body just freezes up. A few times when I just laid there and let him have sex with me, I felt like I was watching him from above. And I can feel some pain, but I can't move. After he is done, he wants to touch me, but I just want to run away.

As we explored this further, she talked about a neighbor who babysat her for a few hours each week for a couple of years from the time she was about seven to nine years old. They had a troubled adolescent son who sexually abused Barb. She said that "it started out with him making me touch him, but he soon made me perform oral sex on him, and then he started to rape me. After each time, he said that if I told anyone, that I would get in trouble, and he would come after me. So, I never said anything."

The abuse was discovered when a teacher noticed Barb scratching her crotch as though she was in pain. The teacher asked her about it and when Barb said that she "itched real bad," the teacher sent her to the school nurse. When the nurse examined Barb, she found a pubic hair in her underwear. The police were called and Barb's parents were notified.

"It was weird, though," Barb said. "It was like my parents just acted like nothing had happened. Growing up, I tried bringing it up to my mom, but she just told me to 'let it go and forget about it.' Throughout high school and college, the only way that I could have sex was if I was drinking a lot. Otherwise I would just freeze up and mentally go somewhere else."

Barb and Rick had a couple of issues that we addressed in therapy. The first was to look at ways to improve the way the two of them engaged each other during times of distress. We worked on techniques that helped them remain emotionally connected with each other during times of conflict. The improved sense of emotional connection between the two of them helped calm Barb's emotions so she didn't become overwhelmed with distress from her interactions with Rick.

The way that Barb's family responded to her sexual abuse in childhood was terrible, but not uncommon. Parents often don't know how to handle their own distress when something bad happens to their kids, so they may either dismiss what had happened, or blame the child in some way. Unfortunately, the way her parents responded left Barb with a sense that no one will be there for her when she is hurt or distressed, which was an emotional trigger for her.

Fortunately, the Rick and Barb were able to make great progress in their ability to communicate with each other, and Rick ended up being a very important part of Barb's recovery from her childhood abuse.

The Crying Valve

The crying valve trauma response is experienced as either the inability to cry, or the inability to stop crying. Crying is an important way for our mind to process grief, and the inability to process grief correctly is due to the way that trauma experiences are processed. This often shows up as the inability to cry in circumstances that would be appropriate, and to cry uncontrollably at times that seem oddly out of place. When I was in graduate school, I remember sitting in one of my trauma classes when this happened to one of my professors. We had been discussing some case studies of people who had experienced various forms of trauma. About ten minutes into the class, one of the students made a comment about a particular case and the entire look on the professor's face changed. She stood there for a moment trying to collect herself as her eyes teared up, and then ran out of the room without saying a word. She never returned to class that day. I could tell what was happening to her because I had experienced something similar several years earlier when I decided to join the Marine Corps.

The Marine in the Hallway

In 1985, I decided to join the Marine Corps in the hope that it would help me get on my feet. I was two years sober at the time and had recently moved out of the abandoned house and into a small apartment that I shared with a woman who was also early in her recovery. In August of that year, I shipped down to Parris Island, South Carolina, to begin what I expected would be a long career in the military. Unfortunately, the emotional trauma I had experienced in childhood ended up derailing that ambition.

One evening, I was sitting on my footlocker in our barracks reading a letter from my father. In the letter, he wrote that his second marriage was "on the rocks." Something happened to me when I read that. I felt my gut wrench tightly and I began to cry uncontrollably—and it wouldn't stop. For a young Marine who was trying to impress everyone with how tough he was, it was not a good look. But, I couldn't help it. I felt like my body was convulsing with an overwhelming mixture of sadness, despair, emptiness, and anguish, and I had no control over what was happening. After about fifteen minutes of this, a drill instructor escorted me into an empty hallway. In a concerned and empathetic tone, he said to come back when I was able. I sat in that hallway and wept hard for over an hour. It may have been two hours. Despite my best efforts to calm myself down, I couldn't. It just had to run its course.

Dissociation

Dissociation is a common experience for most people. It is a way for the brain to engage in creative imagination and disconnect from things that are distressing or tedious, allowing us to disconnect from reality for a bit until circumstances are more interesting and calm. Under normal circumstances, the ability to dissociate allows us to endure long car rides without becoming too distressed from boredom, or emotionally disconnect for a short time when we are in a frightening situation. In a "normal brain," dissociation makes up a small part of our daily experience. However, when someone has experienced trauma, dissociation can become a real problem.

Because emotional trauma keeps us stuck in a state of distress, our brain will tend to dissociate as a coping mechanism. This may lead to a number of symptoms such as the feeling like things are not real or we are living in a dream, having memory lapses about traumatic events or recalling traumatic events in a different chronological order. We may feel separated from life as though we are watching a movie, or may experience a sense of deperaonalization where we feel like we are not ourselves in some way.

Dissociation can also show up as emotional delay where our emotional response to an event doesn't happen until minutes or even hours later when we relive the situation in our head and think of the perfect thing that we should have said. Typically, this is a pattern where you have an emotional freeze response in the moment and don't know what to say or do, followed by an emotional reaction some time later. We also may display emotion that seems inconsistent with what we are saying, such as laughing when describing our trauma or painful situations.

Sitting in the Audience

One of my clients described his experience of dissociation when he first stopped drinking.

> I remember walking alone one night with this feeling like nothing around me was real. It was like I was in a dream, or I was on an alien planet. I felt this odd sense of urgency to keep walking, no matter what, so I just kept walking and walking. Eventually, I came to this winding road next to a river and I sat down. I must have sat there for a couple of hours just watching random cars drive by. It was as though I was sitting in a darkened theater watching cars passing across a movie screen. I just felt so distant and disconnected from it all. In a way, it felt like it wasn't really happening.

The sense of disconnection from what is happening around us is common when someone has experienced emotional trauma, whether it be from assault or abandonment. It is the result of our awareness disconnecting from chronic emotional distress.

The Urgency to Rush to Nowhere

Many people with emotional trauma experience this ill-defined sense of urgency to keep in constant motion. It is as though there is this invisible energy that creates a sense of panic with stillness and routine. This may manifest as a constant change in direction in life, such as shifting career paths every few months to every couple of years, to literally finding it difficult to sit in one place for more than a few minutes.

OUR DYSREGULATED EMOTIONS

Just Go Do Something

One of my clients described how difficult it was for him to sit in lecture during college.

> I remember sitting in the back of the lecture hall feeling like I had to get out of there. It was as if there was some emergency I had to get to. I tried many times to sit through class, but I was only able to do it a few times. The rest of the time, I would just go out to do something. Anything. I would go to a golf driving range, shop at thrift stores, start collecting rocks, just anything that kept me moving and distracted.

He took classes to earn his license as a real estate agent, and before even listing a single house, he changed career directions and got a license to become a stock broker. He then decided that he wanted to pursue a career as a writer, and after starting several books, decided to go back to college to get a degree in business. During all of this, there was this driving sense to "finally find himself" and settle into a routine that would make him feel happy and fulfilled.

This need to keep moving is a common challenge for people with emotional trauma. This is part of the flight response that can happen when trauma memories are recalled. The constant changing of direction and need to keep moving is a way to stay distracted from dealing with the frightening memories and emotions from our traumatic past.

Key Points to Remember

Those of us who have lived with the emotional dysregulation from trauma know firsthand how frustrating and demoralizing it can be. This happens when unprocessed emotional trauma causes your emotional system to be stuck in the fight-or-flight response. One of the goals of recovering from emotional trauma is to shift the brain out of that constant state of distress and into a more calm and balanced state. Some specific tools for doing that will be covered in the Calming Your Emotions chapter.

The key points to remember from this chapter are:

1. There are two parts of our autonomic nervous system: the sympathetic nervous system, and the parasympathetic nervous system. Normally, these two divisions are in balance with each other and will be dominant at different times, depending on whether we are confronting the world or are relaxing.

2. When we experience trauma, our brain becomes stuck in sympathetic dominance and our alarm response can remain activated, even when it should be turned off. This creates a chronic state of stress where our mind and body respond to the world as though they were in a fight for survival.

3. The emotional system being stuck in the alarm response can result a number of trauma-related experiences, including reliving traumatic memories, uncontrolled anger, hypervigilance, reverting to an earlier trauma, emotional numbing, triggering the crying valve, dissociation, and a sense of urgency to rush to nowhere.

All of these are part of the neurological response to trauma in the brain. Healing from this effect of trauma centers around processing trauma memories, calming the nervous system, and attuning our emotional system with the body.

CHAPTER 4

Our Damaged Self-Concept

THOSE OF US WITH emotional trauma will often struggle with a distorted sense of self that can leave us feeling dirty, unsafe, broken, unlovable, unworthy, empty, hopeless, or contaminated in some way. We may feel like a mistake, like we were born on the wrong planet or in the wrong time in history, that there is no goodness in the world, or that we are not normal. We may experience feelings of isolation and alienation, struggle to form and maintain intimate relationships, and may engage in addictive behavior. While we may present ourselves well and even achieve a high level of success, many of us have times when we feel like we are dying inside.

The question is why? What is it about emotional trauma, whether from abuse, neglect, or shaming, that can have such a lifelong impact on our sense of self? If you were sexually molested when you were ten years old, why does it make you feel broken decades later? If your parents emotionally neglected you, why would that still have any impact on you in your thirties, forties, or fifties? If your parents made you feel like you could never do anything right, why would that still affect you now? What is it about this kind of experience that creates such a lasting imprint on the soul? Why can't we just shrug off those experiences as something that happened in the past and move on to a happy and successful life?

The answer is that emotional trauma, particularly during childhood, causes damage to the part of our psyche that I call the "core self-concept." Our core self-concept is responsible for creating a felt sense of being an individual with a coherent identity, whose life is meaningful, of being connected to other people and loved by them, of being safe and secure and able to tackle any challenge you face. When this part of ourselves becomes damaged or doesn't form properly, it can have a lifelong negative impact on how we perceive ourselves and the world around us. It creates a distorted sense of who we are and floods us with distressing emotions that have an impact on our mental and physical health and our ability to form stable intimate relationships.

The Core Self-Concept

Our core self-concept is a deep psychological structure that gives us a sense of being a unique individual and helps us orient to our surroundings. It is like a mental skeleton that gives a basic shape to our psychological and emotional world. It is a scaffolding upon which we build our internal and external boundaries, how we assess danger and our capabilities, and the lens through which we perceive ourselves and understand our place in the world. Our core self-concept is shaped through our experiences related to five critical existential questions:

- Who Am I?
- Am I Alone?
- Am I Safe?

- Am I Loved?
- Can I Affect My World?

The answers to these five existential questions begin to be shaped by our experiences immediately after birth and continue to evolve throughout childhood. The nature of our experiences will determine whether we develop a coherent and stable sense of self or feel lost and rudderless; whether we feel connected to others or isolated and alone; whether we feel secure or fearful; whether we feel empowered or helpless; and whether we feel loved and valued or that life is meaningless and empty. Even before we can speak or understand what is happening around us, our childhood experiences begin to shape our internal model of ourself and the world in which we live. It is like we are born with five empty cups, each with a need that is looking to be filled. Whether those cups are filled or left empty depends on our relationship experiences with our parents and caregivers.

Caregivers Shape Our Core Self-Concept

Our parents and caregivers do more than just provide us with food and shelter to support the development of our physical body. They also play a huge role in how we develop our psychological understanding of ourselves. The special emotional attachment bond that we form with them acts as a mold that shapes our core self-concept and our ability to emotionally attune to ourselves and to others—particularly in intimate relationships.

In his landmark book, *Polarities of Experience*, Sydney Blatt described how every human being confronts two basic psychological developmental challenges throughout their lifetime. The first is to establish and sustain fulfilling attachment relationships, and the second is to create and maintain a coherent and generally positive sense of self. These two dimensions—relationships and the sense of self—develop synergistically with each other. In other words, your sense of self develops through your experiences with attachment relationships, and conversely, how you form attachment relationships with others is heavily influenced by your sense of self. This interdependence between your internal self-concept and your engagement with another in an attachment relationship is an interactive dance between how you experience what is within you (self-concept) and what is between you and your loved one (relationship). Because our self-concept is shaped by our relationship experiences, we need healthy connections with other people in our lives in order to develop a healthy sense of self, and to heal when we are hurt.

The Five Elements of Our Core Self-Concept

In the beginning of this chapter, we discussed the idea that our core self-concept is organized around the five basic existential questions: Who am I? Am I alone? Am I safe? Am I loved? Can I affect my world? There is a part of our primitive emotional system that is very attuned to each of these questions because of their importance to our survival. We live in a dangerous world, and if you are unable to orient yourself to your environment or are abandoned, threatened, unloved, and powerless, you probably aren't going to live very long.

For this reason, any disruption in the development of our sense of identity, feeling connected, feeling safe, feeling loved, and feeling a sense of agency will trigger intense emotional distress. Emotional trauma disrupts our ability to satisfy these five questions in a healthy way. We may struggle to figure out who we are, have difficulty forming relationships, feel anxious and fearful, feel hopelessness and despair, and experience a sense of unlovability.

Let's take a minute to dive a little deeper into each of these five elements of our core self-concept. Understanding these five elements will be very helpful when trying to make sense out of how trauma impacts our experience and how we can heal.

"Who Am I?"
The Need for a Sense of Identity

The term "identity" gets thrown around a lot these days to mean many different things. In our discussion here, we are going to use "identity" in a very specific way. Our identity is the part of us that creates the experience of being present in the world as a unique individual. It creates a sense of boundary that separates us from others and allows us to differentiate between what "is me" and what "is not me," and allows us to maintain a sense of coherence and consistency of who we are when in different situations. It creates a sense of existential orientation that provides us with an intuitive sense of where we fit in the world and what we want to do with our life.

Your Cluster of Parts

We can think about our sense of identity like a cluster of parts connected together into a stable group much like a bunch of grapes. Each one of our "individual grapes" is a part of ourselves that grows out of our central core to meet the needs of a particular circumstance. For example, when we started going to school as a kid, we had to learn how to think, feel, and behave in a school environment. So, we had to develop a new dimension of our identity to meet that challenge. In other words, we grew a new grape, so to speak, that was the student part of ourselves that specialized in meeting the expectations of our role as a student. This new student part may have been a challenge at first, but eventually it became an established part of our identity. It developed into another grape in our cluster that was distinct, but still connected to the other parts of ourselves by a central stem, which was our core sense of self. This part of ourselves was different from the part that helped us engage in play with our friends.

If all went well during our childhood, we developed many parts of ourselves that helped us navigate different situations successfully. In other words, we grew a new grape for each situation to give us an intuitive sense of how to think and act appropriately. As adults, we may have a "job interview" part that acts and thinks very differently than our "party in Vegas" part. We will act and think differently when we are in a business meeting than when we are being intimate with our partner. The part of us that is called into action when we are doing a presentation in front of an audience is different from the part of us that is trying to rescue a cat stuck in a tree, and both of them are different from when we are going to visit a doctor when we are ill. Each of these parts is intended to serve a different function to help us navigate the world effectively. Richard Schwartz, who developed the Internal Family Systems model of psychotherapy, described these parts of ourselves as "not just feelings, but distinct ways of being, with their own beliefs, agendas, and roles in the overall ecology of our lives."

People who have a nontraumatized brain will tend to have a core sense of identity that connects their cluster of parts into a coherent whole. This allows them to easily shift from one part of themselves to another as circumstances change without losing touch with the core sense of who they are. Meanwhile, those of us with a history of emotional trauma will often have a central core that did not form properly or was damaged. So, instead of the parts of ourselves being held together into a coherent cluster by a healthy self-concept, we are often more like a cluster of grapes that are weakly attached to their central stem or have been separated from the other grapes completely. So, we will tend to not have a coherent sense of identity that keeps the parts of ourselves organized into a coherent whole. This can manifest in a couple of ways.

OUR DAMAGED SELF-CONCEPT

For some of us, there are times when our sense of identity can disintegrate into an amorphous cloud where we may feel like our insides are empty, or we don't know what to say or do as though our grapes have disappeared. It is like we just go blank. For others, the opposite may happen and we become rigid, obstinate, and inflexible. It is as though we become stranded on one particular grape and cannot move. In both cases, these responses seem to be particularly prominent during relationship conflict or whenever we are not feeling safe.

The Experience of a Damaged Sense of Identity

Those of us who live with a sense of identity that was either damaged or did not form well during childhood may struggle with some common experiences, such as:

- Feeling like you are easily influenced by other people.
- Feeling like you are always trying to discover and find yourself.
- Feeling like a chameleon who does not fit in.
- Feeling like you are lost or rudderless.
- Feeling like you don't have an intuitive sense of how to act in different situations.
- Feeling like you end up in situations that other people want for you.
- Feeling like you never get to do what makes you happy, or not knowing what would make you happy.
- Feeling like you want to cry when you don't meet others' expectations.
- Feeling a sense of existential disorientation.

- Feeling like you sometimes don't recognize yourself when you look in the mirror.

If you experience these symptoms, it is not because you are inherently flawed or that your brain is broken. In most cases, these feelings are the result of being born with a healthy mind and then growing up in an unhealthy situation where it didn't feel safe to be you. One way that our developing mind dealt with the distress of being shamed, mocked, attacked, molested, or abandoned was to dissociate. That dissociation helped to protect the emotional circuits in our brains from becoming overloaded, but it has the side effect of interfering with the development of our coherence as individuals.

While feeling like you don't have a coherent sense of self can be distressing for sure, it's not a life sentence. We will discuss techniques for strengthening your sense of identity later in the book. For now, I would invite you to just notice whether the symptoms listed above resonate with you.

"Am I Alone?"
The Need for a Sense of Connection

The human brain is one massive organ of attunement that relies on the engagement with others in order to develop and function properly. We all have two major systems of attunement in our brains whose job it is to observe and bond with other people. These are the attachment system and the mirror neuron system. The attachment system seeks to form a special kind of emotional bond between us and our caregivers during childhood, and between us and our partner in adult romantic relationships. Attachment bonds create a sense that our emotional life is tied to the other, as though a part of us exists in their heart, and a part of them exists in ours. This special bond not only makes us feel an intimate connection, but it also serves to regulate our emotions, develops our perception about whether the world is a nurturing or dangerous place, and even shapes our self-concept.

The mirror neuron system is a group of specialized brain cells that fire both when we perform an action and when we observe the same action performed by another. In other words, when we see someone else do something that seems relevant to us, such as interact with others in social situations, talk to us, or cook dinner, our mirror neuron system fires as though we are doing the activity ourselves. The mirror neuron system is why we pick up the behaviors of those around us, how we develop language, how we develop our ability to empathize with others, and may even be the reason why you tend to yawn when you see someone else yawn.

Together, these two attunement systems play an important role in how we develop a sense of self. Experiencing emotional neglect or social isolation can deeply affect us because our brain needs to engage with other people to maintain its health. Solitary confinement is often considered cruel and inhumane punishment because the prolonged isolation leads to the disintegration of the individual's mental and emotional life. This is also why emotionally absent or shaming parents can have such a significant impact on a child's long-term mental and emotional development.

The Effect of Emotional Neglect

Nicolae Ceaușescu, the communist leader of Romania from 1969 to 1985, believed that population growth would lead to the economic growth of the nation, so he instituted a ban on contraception and abortion, encouraged couples to have more babies, and levied a tax on couples who were childless. The ensuing tsunami of babies resulted in roughly five hundred thousand infants and young children being surrendered to orphanages by parents who simply could not afford to raise them. Unfortunately, the government didn't have the resources to support them either, so these children ended up being raised in institutions where they experienced extreme emotional and physical neglect.

The children lived in rows of iron cribs and received very little interpersonal contact. In fact, the nurses were told to limit their contact with the children in order to minimize the risk of spreading illness. Although these children were fed, changed, and occasionally bathed, they received very little emotional connection with their caregivers. The result was that these babies didn't develop normally. They didn't cry when they were distressed or make eye contact with caregivers when fed. They just lay there in a state of dissociation staring blankly into space. Their physical growth was stunted, they didn't develop the ability to speak normally, and they didn't interact with either the other children or adults.

When the condition of these children made international news, there was an enormous response by compassionate families in the United States and Western Europe to adopt these children. When they were adopted, many of these children were in the fifth percentile of physical height, could not communicate, were unable to socialize with other children, and engaged in odd behaviors. The good news is that once these children were in homes where their caregivers actively engaged with them, they rapidly started to develop. Unfortunately, many of them still struggle today with the consequences of the emotional neglect they experienced as children.

Why did this happen? The human brain needs active engagement with others in order for it to develop and function normally. Other people, particularly those close to us, provide a mirror that helps us understand ourselves. When we are upset, others can act as emotional shock absorbers that can help our distressed mind calm down. When we are feeling anxious or afraid, others can help us feel safe and supported. That is, if they are present and emotionally attuned to us.

OUR DAMAGED SELF-CONCEPT

The Experience of a Damaged Sense of Connection

Emotional neglect and isolation are inherently traumatizing because they disrupt our ability to emotionally attune to others. When we are deprived of this critical attunement during childhood, we may experience several problems in adulthood, such as:

- Feeling a sense of internal emotional collapse from perceived rejection
- Becoming hypercritical or aggressive toward our partner or parents
- Feeling a sense of emptiness, loneliness, or boredom
- Struggling with feelings of abandonment
- Feeling like there is some invisible wall that separates us from other people

Again, if you experience some of these things, it is not because you have a broken brain. It is most likely because the experience you had growing up did not provide the level of healthy emotional attunement that allowed that part of your emotional system to develop. Although improving your ability to emotionally attune to yourself and others is harder to achieve in adulthood, it is entirely possible to do. It just takes practice. We will talk about some specific techniques in the chapter Healing Your Core Self.

"Am I Safe?" The Need for a Sense of Safety

Human beings are born in a very immature state and are highly vulnerable to the elements, predators, and disease. Because of this, our brains are highly attuned to perceive and respond to anything that feels threatening to our well-being and will trigger fear whenever it senses danger. This sense of danger does not have to be in the form of a physical threat. Fear can also be triggered from a perceived threat to our emotional connections with others, or feeling rejected, shamed, incapable, or unlovable. In other words, fear will be triggered whenever we perceive some sort of threat to the well-being of our core self. As we discussed in the previous chapter on dysregulated emotion, the fight, flight, freeze, or fawn response tends to be activated whenever we perceive a threat.

The Experience of a Damaged Sense of Safety

Feeling unsafe on occasion is a normal part of living in an unpredictable and often dangerous world. But, if we grow up in a home where we do not feel emotionally or physically safe, or have experienced significant trauma as an adult, we may struggle with some common problems, such as:

- Feelings of dissociation or derealization where it feels like things are not real in some way
- Feeling a sense of panic or discomfort when people become too emotionally close to you
- Feeling a sense of urgency, like you have to get away or rush somewhere
- Struggling with attention and focus, or being diagnosed with ADHD
- Numbing out or freezing when feeling verbally attacked or threatened
- Struggling with episodes of rage that you have trouble controlling
- Laughing when talking about painful things

OUR DAMAGED SELF-CONCEPT

All of these are normal responses to feeling unsafe. Whether we tend to react to a threat with a fight, flight, freeze, or fawn response is not something we can typically choose. A lot of it depends on our experiences growing up, our physical stature, and our personal temperament. When we have to orient our energy toward self-protection, we deprive ourselves of the energy for self-development. When we experience relational trauma growing up, these normal responses to threats may take on a dominant role in our lives and interfere with our ability to respond to others in a healthy way. For example, we may become a people pleaser and find it difficult to set boundaries and get our own needs met because it was not safe for us to do so in our previous relationships with our parents or partners.

"Am I Loved?"
The Need for a Sense of Value

Love is the sense that you are adored and hold a special place of importance in the mind of another human being. It is the sense that another person desires to spend time with you and that they find joy in having you in their life. It is the sense that other people recognize your inherent value and desire to engage with you. It is the feeling that your well-being is important to others and they will make the effort to support you during times of distress. This could be something as simple as going out of their way to be nice when you are in a tough place, or something as extreme as risking their own life to protect yours.

The Root of Self-Esteem

Our self-esteem is rooted in our perceived sense of lovability and value. Self-esteem is a sense that we matter to those around us, we can ask for what we need, and we are deserving of attention and happiness. People with healthy self-esteem tend to be more successful in their relationships and careers because they engage with the world differently than those who feel unlovable.

When our sense of lovability becomes distorted or broken, we will often struggle with feelings of worthlessness, emptiness, or meaninglessness. No matter how many times people may tell us how awesome we are, internally we feel like if they really knew who we were, then they wouldn't like us. This is something that was a struggle for me for much of my adulthood. I remember telling one of my friends many years ago that I could walk into a room where people throw a surprise party for me, sing "For He's a Jolly Good Fellow," and laugh at all of my stupid jokes, and I could still walk out of the room convinced that everyone hates me. Of course, it wasn't true that everyone hated me, but it felt true.

Those who grew up in a home where this critical sense of self was not adequately nurtured will usually enter into adulthood with a sense that they are somehow flawed or deficient. They may find it difficult to accept compliments because the kind words of others feel inconsistent with how they feel about themselves. It is common for people with a damaged sense of value to think things like "if people really knew me, they wouldn't like me," to question why someone would want to be their friend, or to be overly effusive in their gratitude toward people who are kind to them. Lacking an internal sense of worthiness, they may be overly generous with their time, attention, and resources in an unconscious effort to get people to see them as being lovable. They may be drawn to situations that continue to undermine their sense of value, such as remaining in a job, relationship, or activity that is demeaning in some way—often out of some hope that they can win the love of the very people who are incapable of providing it.

OUR DAMAGED SELF-CONCEPT

The Experience of a Damaged Sense of Value

Those of us who live with a damaged sense of value will often struggle with some common experiences, such as:

- Feeling flawed and unlovable
- Feeling like we have to prove our value to others
- Questioning why someone would want to be our friend
- Feeling like our value is based on performance or what we can provide to others
- Struggling with a sense of worthlessness or unworthiness
- Feeling like our needs are a burden to others, or we don't deserve to have our needs met
- Trying to save others and shield them from pain and disappointment

Those of us who grew up in a home where we felt unworthy, unlovable, or that we didn't matter, may find it hard to envision what a healthy self-esteem evem feels like. Since damage to our core self-concept usually begins very early in life, the internalized feelings of unworthiness, deflation, unlovability, and craving for validation may be all we know. We may recite affirmations in an attempt to convince ourselves that we are lovable, but there is often a sense of artifice to it all. More often, we struggle with a nagging sense that we are "just one of those people" that the world has rejected.

As with the other parts of our core self, we can organically develop our sense of lovability in adulthood. It just takes some time and a bond with a loved one. We will discuss specific strategies in the Healing Your Core Self-Concept chapter later in the book.

"Can I Affect My World?" The Need for a Sense of Agency

Agency is the sense that we have control over the events in our lives. It is the sense that we can affect change in the world around us in meaningful ways and that we have confidence that we can successfully navigate through adversity. It is the sense that we can set and reach goals and that our intentional efforts will result in predictable outcomes. It is a sense that we can act effectively in unfamiliar situations and can tolerate some degree of ambiguity. It is the sense that we can set and hold both internal and external boundaries and respond appropriately when those boundaries are violated. It is the sense that no matter what the world throws at us, we will be able to adapt and figure out a way to navigate through it.

The violation of this need for a sense of agency is one of the core elements of a traumatic experience. It is the feeling of being trapped and helpless coupled with extreme distress that leads to the effects of trauma. It is the feeling of being trapped in the airplane as it is going down, feeling physically overpowered during an assault, feeling like you cannot escape from your pain, or feeling like you cannot seem to change your situation no matter how hard you try. In fact, it is this feeling of being trapped and helpless that makes someone suicidal, not just the fact that they are in pain.

The Locus of Control

In 1954, Julian Rotter introduced the concept he called "Locus of Control" as part of his social learning theory, which describes how strongly people believe they have control over the events in their lives. In other words, do I believe that my success or failure is because of my choices, or is it because of external circumstances?

Internal Locus of Control

Those with an internal locus of control believe that they are responsible for their own success or failure. Their actions, efforts, and decisions determine what happens to them. They perceive themselves as having personal control over their behavior, have a greater sense of personal agency, and are more likely to take responsibility for their behavior.

Having an internal locus of control is generally associated with better mental health. People who feel they have a greater sense of agency over their lives tend to experience:

- Lower rates of depression and anxiety
- Higher self-esteem
- Greater resilience to stress
- More proactive coping strategies (e.g., problem-solving instead of avoidance)

External Locus of Control

Those with an external locus of control perceive their circumstances are the result of external influences or luck. Although they may be willing to believe that they may be somewhat at fault, they believe that outside forces, such as luck, fate, or other people, control the outcomes of their life. They are much more likely to blame circumstances for their difficulties, lack a sense of agency, and may reject the idea that their own actions have created their circumstances.

Having an external locus of control is often linked to poorer mental health. People who feel as though they have little sense of agency over their lives tend to experience:

- Higher levels of depression, anxiety, and learned helplessness

- Feelings of hopelessness or powerlessness
- Greater stress, especially in situations that feel uncontrollable
- Passive or avoidant coping styles
- Tendency to hold more hostility and resentment toward others

Locus of control lies on a continuum, and we can feel more on the internal end in some situations and feel more on the external end in others.

The Experience of a Damaged Sense of Agency

Those of us who have experienced a damaged sense of agency will tend to be stuck in the more extreme end of perceiving an external locus of control. We will tend to feel like no matter what we do, we cannot seem to figure out some aspect of our lives. While we may be highly successful and feel fully empowered in some domains of our life, there are others that seem to baffle us. It can be as though we lack an intuitive sense of how to navigate a particular part of our life and may feel frustrated or hopeless. We will explore how to address this later in the book.

Living with a Damaged Core Self-Concept

The holes in the structure of our core self-concept not only deprive us of an intuitive sense of how to successfully navigate through parts of our life that appear effortless to nontraumatized people, but they will also cause us to emotionally react to situations in odd ways. We will tend to misinterpret events in our lives as further evidence of our unlovability or brokenness and respond to that misinterpretation as though it was truth. This is why traumatized people tend to dismiss their own capabilities, feel like nobody loves them when the opposite is true, or feel like they are a failure when they are highly accomplished. Instead of seeing ourselves as intelligent and capable individuals who are valuable and worthy of love, we will tend to see ourselves as broken, dirty, unlovable, or flawed in some way.

Here are some common experiences in those of us who live with the effects of emotional trauma. Depending on your unique experience, who you had as a support system, and your personal temperament, some of these may resonate with you and not others. You may also find that you resonate with all of them.

Inability to Perceive Threats Accurately

Those of us with emotional trauma will often have a hard time perceiving threats accurately. We may perceive a threat where none actually exists, or we may fail to recognize the warning signs of dangerous people and situations. This distortion in perception is the main reason we may feel attracted to unhealthy partners or find ourselves over and over again in situations where we are hurt.

I recall a woman who had come to the Sexual Violence Center back in the 1980s for support following her sixth rape. In every case, she had been hitchhiking alone at night and was picked up by someone who she said "seemed okay." In one of our consultation groups, the director of the center privately said that she felt like slapping the client and yelling, "What the hell were you thinking?" While it would be easy to blame the woman for repeatedly putting herself in the position to be hurt, it is more important to step back from judgment so we can appreciate how her damaged core self-concept from an abusive childhood made it hard for her to recognize warning signs that would have been obvious to others.

On the other side of the coin is the perception of threat where none actually exists. This is often experienced as a sense of panic when someone becomes too emotionally close, or when we view with suspicion those who are trying to be nurturing and supportive. While there may be a part of us that desperately wants to have emotional intimacy, we will tend to push away the people who would love and care for us and instead surround ourselves with others who retreat from emotional closeness.

Feeling Terminally Different

Another very common experience that comes from a broken core self is a persistent and pervasive self-doubt, and the sense that we are not like "normal people." Even when surrounded by friends, we have this sense that somehow other people have some kind of connection with each other that we don't share. We often feel like we are an outsider in some way who may be participating, but is not part of the club. We may feel like things that seem easy for other people are a struggle for us.

There is some truth to our feeling that we are different from "normal people." In some ways we are different. Nontraumatized person can often go through life with a sense of confidence and clarity about who they are and what they want, while those of us with internalized shame are often having to manage self-doubt, anxiety, uncertainty, and dissociation while trying to wear a mask of social acceptability in order to fit in. Unfortunately, the time and energy that we have to devote to maintaining a presentation of normalcy, rather than on our own self-development, often makes success more difficult to achieve.

While those of us who are traumatized can put on a mask of normalcy to get through the day and may be quite successful in some areas of our life, behind the mask many of us carry a sense of emptiness, alienation, and pain that nontraumatized people simply can't understand. At times, being around nontraumatized people can be hard because it just highlights how bad we feel inside.

OUR DAMAGED SELF-CONCEPT

A Sense of Emptiness and Loneliness

One of the ways that this distorted sense of what is real plays out in the lives of many of us who live with emotional trauma, is a sense of emptiness and despair. We may feel that the world lacks any real goodness or kindness. We may feel like our role in life is to be hurt, or that the happiness, love, and success that other people seem to enjoy simply is not for us. We may feel that our life is meaningless, hopeless, and intensely alone.

I received an email one morning from a client who works as on-camera talent for a major media company. He experienced significant relational trauma during childhood, which left him with a deep sense of emptiness and unlovability. Even though he was popular and his audience loved him, behind the scenes, he struggled.

> I woke up again at 2:00 this morning with a painful sense of emptiness. Although I am happily married, and have people in my life who care about me very much, I feel intensely alone. In a few hours, the daylight will break and I will once again put on my mask of confidence and charisma that everyone expects to see. It is a very fine-tuned display carefully crafted through the years to make myself seem worthy of other people's attention, admiration, and love. I am like a great actor who has honed their craft to make the illusion of my character seem very real. I show them a Superman who is motivated and optimistic, and can accomplish anything. During the show, I feel empowered and beloved by the audience, but at some level, I know that they are cheering for the character I portray—not the real me. They are not there to see the lonely and intensely insecure man behind the mask. When the show is over, my mask comes off and the emptiness returns. This is the side of me that I keep hidden from the world. If life has taught me one thing, it's that people love to be entertained, but they will vanish if you take off your mask and expose your soul. The pain of that rejection

is just too intense to bear. So, I go on day after day wearing my mask.

The experience he describes is one that many people with emotional trauma understand. When we are in that space, we may feel like those who are happy and content are just fooling themselves, and that nothing in life matters. Although our feelings are not factually accurate, they feel true.

Seeking Repair from Those Who Cannot Provide It

When we experience emotional trauma from our interaction with someone emotionally bonded to us, there is a natural drive to repair that wound. This is a normal thing to do. The ability to repair the emotional bond with our parents or partners is how stable and fulfilling relationships are able to flourish between imperfect people. However, this only works when both partners participate in the repair. If one person is unable or unwilling to be accountable for their behavior, then repair becomes impossible. One partner cannot repair the relationship for the damage done by the other.

During childhood, the need for a healthy and strong emotional bond with our parents is critical to the development of our sense of self, our ability to self-regulate our emotions, and our ability to form secure emotional bonds as adults. Because of this, children will feel a sense of urgency to reconnect with their parents whenever their parents feel unavailable or are hurtful toward them. Depending on the type of abuse or neglect, we may be very withdrawn and afraid of our parents, or we may act out in order to garner their attention. In either case, there is a deep need for a sense of reconciliation so that we can get our developmental needs met.

OUR DAMAGED SELF-CONCEPT

When we enter into adulthood with emotional trauma from our childhood, we tend to carry with us a deep need for reconciliation and repair from our parents—the people who were unable to provide it in the first place. So, we will tend to engage with our families with this secret hope that maybe this time, things will be different, and they will treat us in a healthier way. We may feel drawn to sacrifice our own priorities or goals and do what will make them happy in the hopes of getting the validation and recognition that we didn't get in childhood. We may feel like we are betraying them in some way, we are abandoning them, or that they will be disappointed in us if we move on and pursue our own hopes and dreams.

This may also play out in how we pick partners. It is common for those of us with emotional trauma to seek out partners with a similar dysfunction as our family of origin. We will tend to gravitate toward those with a relational style that feels familiar to the one in which we grew up. Unfortunately, this usually means that we end up pursuing validation and repair from a partner who is unable to provide it. None of this is rational or intentional. It comes from a deep-seated woundedness that is seeking repair. This is one reason why some people feel drawn to remain in an unhealthy relationship.

Key Points to Remember

Healing your core self-concept is simultaneously the most important and the most difficult part of your recovery journey. It is so critical because without healing our internal sense of self, we will continue to see ourselves and the world around us through a very distorted lens and react to our distorted interpretation as though it was real. This distorted sense of what is real results in our experiencing ourselves in a negative way and reacting to situations in unhelpful ways.

As we transition from childhood to adulthood, we tend to transfer those distorted parts of our core self-concept from our relational space in childhood into the relational space we share with our partners in adulthood. This is both good news and bad news. The bad news is that the emotional baggage and traumas from the relationships we had with our parents that we would love to leave behind us tend to get dragged into our adult relationships, assuming that we are able to successfully maintain relationships at all. The good news is that we can heal our core sense of self in adulthood. Even though we may enter into adulthood with a deep sense of being unlovable and flawed and struggle with relationships, it does not mean that we are trapped in that state for the rest of our lives. People have an amazing capacity to evolve, and can profoundly reshape themselves mentally, emotionally, and physically, if they are willing to step outside of their comfort zone and take the right actions.

In addition to having talent, intelligence, and personality traits, we also have a deeper core sense of self that is responsible for creating our emotional experience of life. Whether we feel happy, fulfilled, and empowered—or sad, empty, and helpless—depends on whether our childhood experiences helped us develop an intact core self. When our core self is healthy, we will experience life as being generally good and meaningful. However, when our core self-concept is damaged, we may struggle with a sense of worthlessness, meaninglessness, unlovability, and hopelessness.

Damage to our core self-concept typically comes from three sources while growing up:

1. Abuse or exposure to violence
2. Emotional neglect
3. Internalized shame

Each of these will affect us differently, but all of them result in a core self that is damaged in some way.

OUR DAMAGED SELF-CONCEPT

The primary effect of damage to our core self-concept is a disconnection between our perception of ourselves and the world with the reality of ourselves and the world. We may feel that people hate us, when they don't. We may feel worthless when, in fact, people value us tremendously. We may feel unlovable when we are surrounded by people who love us. We may feel stuck and hopeless, even when we are making great progress. We may feel afraid and withdraw from the very people who are our biggest allies. But because these distorted perceptions of ourselves are rooted in powerful trauma responses, they feel very real.

In the next chapter, we will discuss how trauma impacts our ability to form and maintain intimate relationships.

CHAPTER 5

Our Difficulties with Relationships

THE STRUGGLE TO FORM healthy and stable intimate relationships is very common in those of us who have experienced emotional trauma. In this chapter, we will talk about how relationships are built on emotional attachment bonds, how disruptions in these attachments in childhood show up in our adult relationships, and how emotional trauma impacts our core sense of self and emotions in a way that makes conflict escalate and more difficult to resolve.

Most of us grew up in homes where we did not have a healthy emotional connection with our parents, and our parents did not have a healthy connection between themselves. So, many of us entered into adulthood without an intuitive sense of what a healthy relationship even looks like. While we may be acutely aware of what it's like to be in a dysfunctional family and don't want to repeat those patterns in our own relationships, we often struggle to do things in a healthier way. Not only did patterns of violence, abuse, emotional neglect, or growing up in a dysfunctional environment impact how we experience emotions and distort the development of our core self-concept, it also affected our ability to successfully form stable and secure attachment bonds.

Growing up in an unhealthy environment led to us developing some coping strategies to help us deal with not getting our emotional needs met. While those coping strategies helped us adapt to an unhealthy family system so that we could function when we were children, they can get in the way of our ability to form and maintain healthy emotional connections as adults. Unless we intentionally focus our energy on breaking dysfunctional ways of relating, we may end up repeating some of the same dysfunctional patterns in our own relationships that we observed in our parents.

The good news is that our past does not have to equal our future. We can learn how to form healthy emotional bonds with our partners today, even if we did not have them while we were growing up. We just need to learn new skills to help us form healthier emotional attachment bonds and to navigate through conflict in a healthier way. Let's start by taking a closer look at emotional attachment bonds.

Emotional Attachment Bonds

An attachment bond is much like a partial fusing of the soul that connects the emotional lives of each person in the relationship and creates a unique sense of completion and wholeness. It is as though each holds the presence of the other in their heart. These emotional connections are like a gravitational force that serves to organize the emotional lives of each person into a stable orbit around the other. It is this bond that creates the sense of togetherness, being loved, and feeling supported. It insulates each person from the terror of isolation, calms the emotional systems in the brain, and can even reduce the sensation of pain. It is the center of the interpersonal universe that fulfills a very primal drive for connection and plays a central role in our psychological and emotional health both as children and adults.

OUR DIFFICULTIES WITH RELATIONSHIPS

In childhood, attachment bonds form a critical connection between children and their primary caregivers. It creates a secure base upon which children develop their understanding of themselves and the world around them. Attachment bonds not only help ensure the physical survival of the child, but also direct the development of their core sense of self and their ability to emotionally self-regulate. This second function is perhaps the most relevant when it comes to our relationships and emotional well-being. The way in which we formed attachment bonds with our caregivers as children has a profound influence on how we form relationships in adulthood and whether the general theme of our emotional life is one of self-compassion or self-shame.

Attachment bonds in adulthood serve many of the same purposes as they do in childhood, but they differ in one important way. While childhood attachment bonds are dependent relationships, where the child is completely dependent on their caregiver for nurturing and support, adult attachments are interdependent relationships where each partner mutually provides nurturing and support for the other. They are the secure base upon which couples build their lives together and move through life as a team.

Unfortunately, most of us who have experienced emotional trauma while growing up will have an attachment style that can get in the way of our ability to connect to our partner, particularly during times of conflict. Depending on the type of attachment injury we experienced, we may find ourselves feeling anxiety about rejection and abandonment, being uncomfortable with intimacy, or having relationships that are unstable and chaotic. Understanding how our early attachment injuries shape our attachment style as adults is helpful in identifying unhealthy patterns in our intimate relationships.

The Four Attachment Styles

There are four basic types of emotional attachment that form between children and their caregivers, depending on the nature of their relationship: secure, anxious, avoidant, and disorganized. Let's take a quick look at each of them.

Secure Attachment

Securely attached children don't seem to experience a lot of anxiety about being abandoned, so they tend to be less fearful when a parent is absent. They like being close to a parent and find it comforting, so these kids tend to approach parents for comfort and connection whenever they are distressed. Children with a secure attachment style tend to seek out comfort from others during periods of difficulty, and they will be more confident venturing out to experience new things. Securely attached kids tolerate being away from their parents fairly well, so spending the night at a friend's house or going camping with a group is not a distressing experience for them. They tend to smile and feel joy when reuniting with their parents after a period of absence, make and retain friendships with peers easily, and tend to do better in school than those with anxious or disorganized attachment.

Securely attached adults experience their relationships as stable and fulfilling. They will tend to feel the presence of the other, even when separated for a time, and find joy and comfort when being together. Mutual nurturing and caregiving allows them to find comfort in their partner during times of distress, and they can develop a deep sense of trust. When faced with difficulties, securely attached adults are able to collaborate and work through issues with their partner and are able to repair their sense of connection after a conflict.

Anxious Attachment

Anxiously attached children tend to experience anxiety about being abandoned, so they tend to be distressed with the absence of their parents. Like the securely attached kids, they are comforted by being close to a parent, so they also approach parents for comfort and connection. However, children with an anxious attachment style have a tendency to act clingy toward their parents, and often experience distress with separation. They may be inconsolable during a parent's absence and often struggle to self-soothe their emotions. It is not uncommon for anxiously attached kids to lash out verbally or physically toward their parent as a way of protesting their absence.

Anxiously attached adults will tend to have a deep fear of abandonment. An anxious partner will tend to urgently pursue the attention of the other and will tend to become aggressive or shaming for any perceived unavailability or abandonment. Anxious partners will tend to experience more jealousy and paranoia about their partners being unfaithful. Unlike couples with secure attachment, they will struggle to effectively repair after conflict and will tend to have the same pattern of conflict over and over again.

Avoidant Attachment

Avoidantly attached children don't experience anxiety when separated from a parent, and don't really seem all that interested in connecting with them when the parent is around. If anything, they experience closeness as distressing, so they tend to simply avoid connection. Children with an avoidant attachment style will often appear checked out from what is going on with their parents. Whether the parent is present or not does not seem to matter much to the child. It's as though they are just one of many adults who are part of their lives. Many of these kids exist in a state of semi-dissociation and retreat into an internal world where they emotionally detach from those around them.

Adults with an avoidant attachment style will tend to struggle to maintain emotional connection, particularly during times of conflict. The most common scenario is a couple who struggle because one partner emotionally shuts down and disengages from the relationship whenever they perceive the other partner becoming critical or angry. If we could peek into the soul of the avoidant partner, we typically would see a partial disintegration of their sense of self during periods of relationship distress. It is as though a part of themselves devolves into an amorphous and diffuse state where there is no clear sense of what is being experienced. When asked to describe what they are feeling, people in this state may look inward and not see anything recognizable. It's like looking into fog. There is often nothing but an ill-defined sense of not being okay and feeling "numbed out." They will often say that they have no idea what they are feeling, and when pressed, may only be able to describe vague sensations such as feeling tense, a pressure in their gut, or as if they are shut down.

Disorganized Attachment

Children with disorganized attachment are like anxiously attached kids in that they tend to experience a lot of distress when separated from their parent, but they are also like the avoidant attached kids who actively avoid closeness with their parents. Children with a disorganized attachment style are in a real tough spot because they are stuck between feeling a sense of panic from being separated from their parent, and a terror of being close. This kind of conflict tends to result from growing up in abusive, chaotic, violent, or alcoholic families, where their parents are simultaneously the source of comfort and pain. Children with a disorganized attachment style may develop an incoherent sense of self and experience significant dissociation.

Adults who have a disorganized attachment style tend to be the most unstable and unpredictable, and their relationships tend to be rife with unresolved conflict. They will tend to struggle with a simultaneous fear of closeness and fear of abandonment. So, they tend to have a chaotic orientation toward their partner that swings between a strong desire for closeness and acting aggressively toward them. At the core of this kind of relationship is a partner who was very wounded in childhood. Most often, people with this attachment style grew up in homes marked by shame-based parenting, a chaotic home life, narcissistic parents, and inconsistent parenting that was very disorienting. Because of this, their attachment style tends to be disoriented, chaotic, and unstable.

Emotional Trauma and Patterns of Conflict

For those of us who have experienced emotional trauma, we may find ourselves stuck in patterns of conflict that never seem to be resolved. Despite the fact that we may get along great with our partner most of the time, there are other times when it seems like conflict escalates and takes on a life of its own. It is like something takes over the conversation and sets us on a destructive path of interaction that ends when someone becomes violent, emotionally shuts down, or walks away in frustration. During these times, we may feel overwhelmed, rageful, dismissed, defensive, alone, numb, or have an urgency to run. We may say things to our partner or act out in hurtful ways that seem extreme or out of context. Rarely does there ever seem to be any resolution or repair. Instead, we just learn to stuff it away and move forward as though nothing had happened.

Unfortunately, the pattern of unresolved conflict and lack of emotional repair results in us building up layers of emotional scar tissue over time that makes us feel even more distant. Repeated cycles of unresolved conflict erodes our emotional connection with our partner and sets up a dynamic where we will tend to avoid certain conversations to avoid triggering another fight. This can feel incredibly frustrating to both partners. While couples may function very well together in so many areas of their life, why is it that certain things tend to trigger emotionally intense arguments that escalate out of control?

The answer, in most cases, is that something in the way the partners interact with each other triggers an emotional trauma response in one or both partners. Once a trauma response enters into the conversation, the energy behind the disagreement has little to do with the topic at hand and more to do with our emotional wounds. Unless we have the ability to recognize when a trauma response enters the conversation, the conflict will tend to escalate, both partners become more emotionally dysregulated, and unhelpful attachment behaviors start to show up. So, a simple conversation that may have started out as a calm discussion about what to do for the holidays can quickly escalate into a fight that seems impossible to resolve.

Conflict Patterns and Your Self-Concept

In the previous chapter, we discussed how each of us has five basic existential needs that organize our core self-concept:

- The need for a sense of identity
- The need for a sense of connection
- The need for a sense of safety
- The need for a sense of value
- The need for a sense of agency

Because these five needs are tied to very primitive survival circuits in the brain, we will tend to react strongly when one or more of these is threatened. For someone who has never experienced emotional trauma, having a conversation about vacation plans, deciding who to invite for dinner, or whether the kids should be involved in certain activities at school doesn't typically trigger a perceived threat to their sense of self. However, for those of us who have experienced damage to our core sense of self from our experiences growing up, it's a different story. Because wounds to our core sense of self distort the way we perceive our interactions with others, we may feel unheard, invalidated, unloved, unsafe, abandoned, helpless, and distressed by things that our partner says or does—things that may not have triggered those same feelings in someone who has a nontraumatized brain. It doesn't mean that our feelings are not real. It just means that we have to be aware of how our own perceptions may be influenced by our emotional trauma.

Conflict patterns in our relationships tend to mirror the woundedness of each partner. For example, partners with a wounded sense of value will tend to perceive interactions through the lens that they don't matter. They will tend to be very sensitive to feeling unheard, unwanted, or unlovable. Partners with a wounded sense of safety will tend to be very sensitive to any implication of emotional or physical threat and may tend to perceive that everyone is against them. Partners with a wounded sense of connection may be very sensitive to any implication of abandonment or that their partner will leave them, and may experience jealousy or distress from any perceived shift of attention away from them.

The main point here is that something in the conversation triggers a trauma response from our wounded core sense of self. In fact, we can get a good sense of where our personal woundedness lies simply by observing what tends to trigger us. When the wounds to our core self become triggered, the alarm response becomes activated in an attempt to cope with the perceived threat to our well-being.

Emotional Inflection Points

Most of us have experienced being in a conversation with someone that was going well, and then suddenly the tone of the conversation seemed to shift into being more emotionally charged. What may have started out as a calm discussion turned into a tense or adversarial exchange where we suddenly felt at odds with each other. If we could go back in time and replay the conversation slowly, we invariably find a moment in time when the tone shifted. There was something that was said or some gesture that seemed to mark the moment when the tone of the conversation changed. I call those moments of change inflection points.

An inflection point is a moment in a conversation when a trauma response is triggered in one or both of the partners, and the emotional shift from the trauma response will be felt as a change in the emotional tone of the conversation. Because these inflection points often arise from emotional trauma, not only will the emotional tone change, but so will how each partner perceives the situation, and how they interact with each other. Once the emotional state of one or both partners begins to flood with dysregulated emotion and the alarm response becomes activated, the conflict will actually no longer be about the topic of the original conversation. It will center around an unmet need to feel heard, safe, validated, empowered, or valued. As long as the partners continue arguing over the original topic, rather than addressing these unmet needs, the argument will tend to continue to escalate.

The Alarm Response

As we talked about in the chapter on dysregulated emotions, the alarm response, also known as the fight, flight, freeze, or fawn response, is a pattern of emotional, physiological, and behavioral responses that are designed to help us cope with a perceived threat to our well-being. When these perceived threats are experienced in a relationship, they can lead to patterns of conflict or disengagement that make it very difficult for partners to remain present with each other. This is because the alarm response is designed to separate us from a perceived threat. When that perceived threat is our partner, it leads to us emotionally disconnecting from them. Let's take a quick look at some of the ways these can show up.

The Fight Response

If we go into the fight response we will tend to engage in angry, shaming, or passive-aggressive behavior toward our partner. This is more common in someone who has an anxious or disorganized attachment style. This may show up as making verbal demands and being hypercritical, sarcastic, dismissive, or aggressive. Even when saying mean things, the intent of the person in fight mode is usually not to be hurtful; they are trying to get their partner to see them, understand them, and validate them. Unfortunately, their aggression and communication style work against the very thing that they are seeking to experience: feeling safe, validated, and that their partner is present.

His Late Flights

Brian and Nancy had been married for about ten years when they came in to see me. Brian worked as an airline pilot and Nancy had an administrative position that allowed her to work from home. She had experienced emotional neglect while growing up that left her with an intense reaction to perceived abandonment. This played out in their marriage by her becoming very angry with him whenever Brian had longer flights where he would not arrive home until later in the evening. When he was working the later flights, Nancy would intentionally put the children to bed early before Brian got home so he couldn't wish them good night, and would not cook any dinner for him when she cooked dinner for the rest of the family so he had nothing to eat when he arrived home. In fact, in one of our sessions, she turned to him and angrily snapped, "Don't expect me to have dinner for you when you get home!" When Brian did get home, she would verbally attack him for seemingly arbitrary and minor things that happened throughout the day when "he should have been there." She didn't act the same way toward him when he arrived home early; only when he had late flights.

It was critical to help her identify how her own experience with relational trauma growing up was triggering her feelings of abandonment. Until she could heal that part of her core sense of self that was previously damaged in childhood, it was difficult for her to be emotionally present in the relationship. Once we addressed some of those trauma issues in the context of couple therapy, they were better able to remain emotionally connected with each other, and their relationship dramatically improved.

The Flight Response

A person in the flight response will tend to emotionally shut down and withdraw from their partner during conflict. This is more common in someone with an avoidant attachment style. Outwardly, it may look like they are disinterested, don't care, or are checking out, but emotionally, people in flight mode feel overwhelmed and shut down. During times of conflict, they may feel like they can never do anything right, and feel inadequate, frustrated, and like a failure. They may feel as though they are emotionally collapsing on the inside where everything feels overwhelming and catastrophic. They may deflect or discredit what their partner is saying in an attempt to deflect criticism.

OUR DIFFICULTIES WITH RELATIONSHIPS

Sitting in His Car

Trevor and Rita came to see me after years of struggling with a repetitive pattern of conflict that left them both feeling hopeless and alone. Rita worked as a psychologist for a school district and Trevor was a construction supervisor. They had been married for fifteen years, had three children, and both of them commented that the other partner was a great parent who was very engaged with their children, and that they often would have several weeks where they got along great and had no issues at all. But then they would fall into an intense cycle of conflict where Rita would become very verbally critical and shaming of Trevor, and Trevor would emotionally shut down and walk away—often going to the garage and just sitting in his car until "things blew over."

When we dug deeper to understand what caused them to shift into a pattern of conflict after doing so well, Rita shared that she would originally become triggered after Trevor said that he would do something and then didn't follow through. During those times, she perceived that to mean that Trevor didn't care about her, and she felt herself fill with a sense of rage. When Trevor sensed that Rita was upset with him, a whole narrative would start playing out in his head that he was a failure, that he could never do enough, that it was his fault that she was upset, and that he could never do anything right. This triggered an internal emotional collapse where he just shut down emotionally. As Rita's anger increased, he felt an urgency to escape and walked away to go sit in his car until his own trauma response calmed down.

It was pretty clear from their pattern that Rita had an anxious attachment style and Trevor had an avoidant attachment style. So, we had to explore more effective ways for Rita to communicate when she felt that Trevor was not there for her that didn't involve anger and criticism, and how Trevor could remain present with Rita's distress so that she didn't feel like he abandoned her whenever she was upset. By implementing some of the tools outlined later in this book, they were able to evolve away from their unhealthy pattern of conflict.

The Freeze Response

A person in the freeze response will tend to dissociate and lose the integrity of their sense of self during conflict. Outwardly, they may look like they are in the flight response because they become quiet and disengaged, but on the inside the experience is quite different. Where someone in the flight response will emotionally shut down and withdraw from engagement, someone in the freeze response will go into a state of panic where a part of themselves just evaporates into an amorphous cloud. When in this state, it is like the ability to think, feel, or respond goes offline, and they may stand there frozen not knowing what to say or do.

Evaporating on the Inside

A couple I worked with early in my practice was a perfect example of this. One of the partners, Keith, grew up with an intense feeling of isolation and constant shaming from his parents. To cope with the distress of chronic loneliness and shaming, he learned to dissociate from his emotions. Now in an adult relationship, he really struggled to remain emotionally present. Whenever he and his partner John had a disagreement, Keith felt himself go numb and silent. When we slowed things down to explore what was happening to him, he described an experience of feeling like he "evaporates inside" whenever John became upset. "It's like my insides just go 'poof' into a cloud of smoke," he said. We referred to that in our sessions as him "poofinating" during times of distress. It was funny, but it worked. When he went silent during a session, I would ask him if he was "poofinating," and most of the time that was exactly what was happening to him. This was a valuable insight because it helped John understand why Keith sometimes went silent during a disagreement, and we could talk about what to do when it happened.

The key to helping Keith remain more present in disagreements with John, was to give them both some non-shaming language that they could use to avoid triggering Keith's "poofinating," and have Keith start some embodiment exercises to help him remain emotionally present. Over time, this helped them break out of their cycle and develop a more effective communication style where both of them felt present and heard.

The Fawn Response

A person in the fawn response will tend to suppress their own distress and seek to soothe the distress in their partner as a way to gain approval, love, or a sense of safety. This is more common in those with a disorganized attachment style. By making themselves more likable to an emotionally dysregulated partner, they hope to reduce the likelihood that they will be the target of aggression. This is more common in those who grew up in unsafe or violent homes where they had to learn to read emotional cues very closely and to shape their behavior to minimize the risk of harm. Over time, fawning becomes an automatic way to navigate relationships, often leading to codependency or difficulty asserting boundaries in adulthood.

Big Mike

I recall a couple who came to see me for one visit many years ago. From the moment they stepped into my office, they just exuded an intense feeling of dysfunction and sickness. I do not often immediately dislike anyone who comes into my office, but that was not the case with "Big Mike." He strutted in wearing a biker jacket and acted like an arrogant jerk. It was clear that he didn't want to be in therapy, but was told by a judge to seek therapy following a recent arrest for domestic violence. His wife, Carol, was thin and pretty with long blond hair and a big smile that stood in stark contrast to Big Mike's burly physique, grungy clothing, intense look, and scruffy beard. As the conversation unfolded, I noticed a couple of interesting things. Big Mike hardly said a word. When I would ask him a direct question, Carol jumped in to answer it for him. For example, when I asked him what had happened the night he was arrested, Carol said that they had a disagreement and that the police didn't need to arrest Big Mike. When I asked her to let him answer, she had a hard time staying quiet. After Big Mike would say a word or two, she would interrupt to defend him.

As I observed Carol, there seemed to be something off in the way she spoke. She made light of the situation and smiled a lot as if to sell me on the idea that nothing bad was happening. He just looked at me the whole time with an uninterested expression on his face as if he was just trying to get through the next fifty-five minutes so his attorney could tell the judge that he saw a therapist. Carol, on the other hand, was quite animated. She seemed jittery and nervous, and even laughed a couple of times when talking about the night Big Mike was arrested. But something in her eyes told me a different story. She had this tension around her eyes that made her look like she was terrified and desperate.

Toward the end of our session, I asked Big Mike to step out for a moment and wait in the reception area. I asked Carol what was going on and whether she felt safe. She assured me that everything was fine, but her demeanor suggested otherwise.

Pulling It All Together

So far we have discussed how attachment bonds form the connection between partners and how attachment styles from childhood can show up in adult relationships. We discussed how our patterns of conflict tend to be organized around injuries to our core sense of self, and why conflict tends to escalate when our emotional trauma responses become triggered. We also discussed how the fight, flight, freeze, or fawn response affects how we react to distress within our relationships. I know that I have presented a lot of material here.

Our next step is to pull all of this information together to help us gain some clarity on how to identify problem areas in our relationships and have some insight on whether we are in a functional relationship, are in a relationship that is struggling, or whether we are in a toxic relationship. With this information, we can develop a strategy for how to move forward in a positive way for both ourselves and our ability to connect with our partners.

Functional, Struggling, and Toxic Relationships

Over the years, I have come to look at relationships as being in one of three categories: relationships that are functional, relationships that are struggling, and relationships that are toxic. We will talk about what each of these categories mean and what constitutes a functional relationship versus one that is struggling or toxic. But first, I think it is important to make a couple of points.

The first is that your attachment style does not define whether your relationship is functional or not. There are plenty of people with anxious, avoidant, or disorganized attachment styles that are able to form stable emotional bonds with their partners and have perfectly functional relationships. Where the difference in attachment style comes into play is the way in which you tend to respond to distress in the relationship. Those with an anxious attachment style will tend to become more critical of their partner, those with an avoidant attachment style will tend to shut down, and those with a disorganized attachment style may do either. Being able to identify when your attachment style is affecting your ability to remain present with your partner will make it easier for you to employ some new skills to help you remain present.

The second is that how trauma responses from your wounded core sense of self show up in your relationship also does not define whether you have a functional relationship or not. There are many people who struggle with significant emotional trauma who are able to form and maintain healthy relationships when they learn how to identify when their trauma responses are being triggered and learn new ways of navigating through the emotions that come up.

The third is that how the fight, flight, freeze, or fawn response shows up in your relationship also does not define whether you have a functional relationship or not. As we discussed earlier, there are many people who tend to go into a freeze response, or a flight response, or a fawn response, or a fight response, when they feel threatened, but they are still able to have a perfectly functional relationship. It is all about developing an awareness of when that response emerges and learning how to navigate through it more effectively.

What really defines the differences between functional, struggling, and toxic relationships are five things:

- The ability to repair after conflict
- The ability to evolve after conflict
- The ability to be mutually supportive
- The ability to communicate effectively
- The ability to have emotional awareness

Let's take a look at how each of these five elements define the quality of the relationship.

Functional Relationships

These couples have the "mythical functional relationship" that many claim doesn't exist. But I can assure you that it does. A functional relationship is simply a securely attached relationship where the partners have a stable emotional bond, where there is mutual caregiving, where they can overcome challenges in a collaborative way, and where they can repair their connection after conflict. That's it. Functional couples are not perfect. They may still argue at times, but they have the ability to emotionally reconnect, repair hurt feelings, and ultimately find a way to work collaboratively. Over time, the ability to navigate conflict effectively serves to deepen their sense of connection and resilience.

The Ability to Repair after Conflict

In functional relationships, couples have the ability to repair after conflict. Although they may have to step away from each other for a time, they are able to reconnect and process through what happened. This typically includes each partner taking accountability for their part in the conflict. For example, while one partner may clearly be the major offending party, as in the case of a violation of trust, the other partner may respond in ways that undermine the couple's ability to repair. Each partner will have the ability to share their emotional experience with the other in the moment, which allows them to emotionally re-attune to each other, and they will be able to express their love and support for each other.

The Ability to Evolve after Conflict

Couples in functional relationships will have the ability to evolve, so they don't often become stuck in repetitive patterns of conflict. They are able to discuss how to avoid a particular conflict in the future, and each partner will change their behavior to be present in a more positive way. The ability to evolve after conflict allows a couple to develop a deeper sense of connection and trust with each other over time and will tend to experience less distress when conflict does arise.

The Ability to be Mutually Supportive

Couples in functional relationships are able to shift between being nurtured by their partner and being a caregiver for their partner. This ability to shift back and forth as the need arises allows both partners to feel supported and engaged in the well-being of the relationship. This in turn provides a conduit through which emotional healing can take place from events outside of the relationship, such as grieving a loss, stress at work, or even the effects of childhood trauma.

The Ability to Communicate Effectively

Couples in functional relationships have the ability engage in communication that helps partners to attune to each other because they often grew up in homes where good communication skills were modeled by their parents. Even if their parents did not model good emotional communication, partners in functional relationships will typically have done some personal work to improve the way they communicate with their partners.

The Ability to Be Emotionally Aware

Couples in functional relationships tend to have good emotional awareness and have the ability to communicate it to their partner in an accurate way.

Struggling Relationships

In many respects, struggling relationships are not that different from functional relationships. In fact, even relationships that are marked by unresolved conflict and emotional disconnection have partners that do most things right most of the time. The big difference between functional relationships and struggling relationships is their inability to repair after conflict, their inability to evolve, and their inability to effectively communicate. Over time, struggling couples may lose a sense of intimate connection and give up on trying to restore it.

The Struggle to Repair after Conflict

One of the hallmarks of a struggling relationship is one marked by escalating conflict with the difficulty in repairing after the conflict ends. As we discussed earlier, this is often because of the way emotional trauma becomes triggered during conflict and causes both partners to emotionally dysregulate. This often leaves both partners feeling a sense of hopelessness, isolation, and frustration.

The Struggle to Evolve after Conflict

When trauma responses become involved in conflict, they have the effect of keeping a couple stuck in a repeated pattern. This happens because unresolved trauma is, by definition, anchored in past experience and will tend to be reexperienced over and over again. The difficulty of moving on and stop repeatedly having the same argument can become a big source of frustration for a struggling couple.

The Struggle to Be Mutually Supportive

Couples who are struggling often will be able to be mutually supportive to each other most of the time. However, once some disagreement emerges, their ability to remain supportive is lost and they feel a shift from collaboration to being adversarial toward each other.

The Struggle to Communicate Effectively

Couples who are struggling tend to engage in communication strategies that push each other away, rather than draw each other close. This is especially true during conflict. Because much of the conflict in struggling couples is driven by emotional trauma and insecure attachment styles, their communication tends to reinforce their trauma response.

The Struggle to Be Emotionally Aware

Couples who are struggling tend to have at least one partner who has difficulty with emotional awareness or emotional communication, particularly during times of distress. This affects their ability to be emotionally present with their partner and can trigger unhelpful emotional responses in their partner.

Toxic Relationships

Toxic relationships are different from both functional and struggling relationships in important ways. The first is that the relationship often has one partner who struggles with an active addiction or a personality disorder, such as narcissistic, antisocial, borderline, or histrionic personality disorders. I call these "toxic partners" because of the damaging impact that their poor emotional awareness, extreme self-orientation, and lack accountability has on the relationship and the emotional life of their partners. Toxic partners are not necessarily bad people. In fact, they may be very charismatic, successful, and well-liked in other areas of their life. But in the context of attachment relationships, their woundedness keeps them from being able to form healthy attachment bonds. Toxic relationships differ from functional and struggling relationships in a few important ways.

OUR DIFFICULTIES WITH RELATIONSHIPS

The Inability to Repair after Conflict

Couples in a toxic relationship typically cannot repair after a conflict. This is due to the difficulty that toxic partners have in personal accountability. The externalization of blame from a toxic partner usually results in their partner having to do all the emotional work of suppressing their own hurt feelings to restore emotional stability.

The Inability to Evolve after Conflict

Couples in toxic relationships struggle to evolve after conflict because one or both partners often lack the ability to evolve themselves. Therefore, cycles of conflict tend to repeat in predictable patterns that only seem to become worse over time, until the toxic partner begins to heal themselves.

The Inability to Be Mutually Supportive

Toxic partners lack the ability to be emotionally available or supportive and are very emotionally needy. For this reason, the nontoxic partner often ends up having to suppress their own needs for support in order to satisfy the needs of the toxic partner. Over time, the nontoxic person often becomes emotionally burnt out.

The Inability to Communicate Effectively

Partners in toxic relationships tend to engage in unhealthy communication. Instead of both partners being able to communicate authentically, there is a lot of manipulation and deception. Toxic partners often cannot tolerate being challenged or hearing how their behavior is affecting others, so communication is often crafted in a way to avoid triggering them.

The Inability to be Emotional Aware

Often, neither partner in a toxic relationship has a good sense of emotional awareness. The toxic partner is typically dissociated from their emotional state, so they are unaware of what they are experiencing. The nontoxic partner often dissociates from their own emotions as a survival strategy, but may be very attuned to cues regarding what the toxic partner is experiencing. Without emotional awareness, the partners are unable to create a functional relationship.

Key Points to Remember

All relationship problems are caused by one thing: something in the way partners interact with each other undermines their ability to remain emotionally connected, particularly during times of distress or conflict. When they are upset and reach out to each other, their pattern of interaction ends up pushing each other away. Although couples do this in different ways, the end result is the same. They engage in a destructive pattern of communication that leaves both of them feeling frustrated and alone.

Difficulty in creating and maintaining these bonds often starts very early in our childhood when our emotional attachment to our parents is disrupted in some way. Disrupted childhood attachment bonds not only impact the emotional system in our brain and the core self, but also the way in which we form attachment bonds in adulthood. This is why so many people who experienced emotional trauma struggle with relationships as adults.

In most couples, these unhelpful patterns can be understood as a type of trauma response. Trauma responses are emotional adaptations to dysfunctional environments or extremely stressful events that impact our sense of self and our ability to emotionally self-regulate. They have a disorganized and destabilizing effect on the relationship that undermines the partners' ability to attune to each other in an organized and healthy way. While trauma is not the cause of all relationship problems, virtually all people with trauma will struggle to form and maintain intimate relationships due to the dysregulated nature of their emotions, disruption in their sense of self, and insecure attachment style.

Emotional trauma triggers can come out of nowhere and may seem off-point or disproportionate to the situation. Because of the nature of unresolved trauma, feelings from previous events or arguments may also be pulled into a present argument, often resulting in conflict spiraling out of control and with no solution in sight. Our damaged core self will also complicate matters as feelings of abandonment, shame, worthlessness, and helplessness get pulled into an already dysregulated communication cycle. This can lead to partners becoming hypercritical of the other or just emotionally shutting down completely.

The final point that is important to know is that relationships can evolve from struggling or toxic relationships into functional ones. It all depends on whether both partners are willing and capable of stepping outside their comfort zone and take the necessary action to change.

CHAPTER 6

The Holistic Healing Mindset

EVERYTHING THAT WE HAVE discussed so far illustrates one important point: emotional trauma is a corroding thread that becomes woven into the fabric of our existence and seems to affect everything. It affects how we think, feel, and act, and even impacts the health of our physical body. Because of this, taking a holistic approach as we navigate our journey going forward will be the most effective way to heal from the wounds of our past. The word *holistic* simply means that we want to heal all parts of ourselves simultaneously in an intentional and coherent way to maximize the benefits we experience from our efforts. We want to create a path forward that will help us heal mentally, emotionally, physically, sexually, and spiritually, so that we can become the fully integrated and vibrant individuals that we were meant to be.

In the upcoming chapters, we will explore ways to calm our emotions, heal our core self-concept, and strengthen our relationships so that we can improve our experience in every dimension of life. But first, let's discuss how to create a holistic healing mindset to help you be successful in your journey. This is based on what I call the Ten Principles of Recovery.

The Ten Principles of Recovery

The Ten Principles of Recovery are simple ideas about how to approach healing from emotional trauma. These are principles that I have discovered through trial and error and a lot of hard work. They helped me in my own healing journey and have proven to be key to helping many of my clients make good progress. These are not healing techniques, but rather a general approach to recovery.

1. The Gift Is in the Grind

Recovering from emotional trauma takes time. It does not happen overnight. Most of us have been living with the effects of emotional trauma for quite some time and we often have a sense of urgency to feel better as quickly as possible. I totally understand that feeling, but we have to give ourselves some time to heal.

We can think of our healing journey like an exercise and weight loss program. We don't expect that we can eat a salad and hit the gym a few times and suddenly go from being overweight and sedentary to looking like a fitness model. That's just not how the body responds. To transform our physical body, we need to apply sustained effort over time. If we do this, then we can transform how we physically look and feel. Even more importantly, by going through the process of changing our focus to living in a more healthy way, we transform who we are as people. In other words, how we physically look as a result of focusing our attention on a healthier life is less important than who we become as individuals by going through the process. As anyone who is in great shape will tell you, there is no point where you ever "arrive" and don't have to exercise anymore. Living a healthy lifestyle is a process, not a destination.

The same is true with our emotional healing journey. Recovery is not a destination to be reached, but a pattern of living to be sustained over time. Achieving success in the future is simply a repetition of success in the moment. As my good friend and mentor Mark LeBlanc says, "The gift is in the grind." Momentum in our healing journey is achieved by focusing on the next right step over and over again. It is a way we live our life. If we approach our recovery like a lifestyle, rather than an outcome, we are far more likely to wake up one day and realize how far we have come. By focusing on small wins in the moment, we also avoid setting ourselves up for disappointment for not reaching some arbitrary and unrealistic goal that we set for ourselves.

2. Your Past Does Not Equal Your Future

Just because we have suffered from the effects of trauma from our past, does not mean that we have to continue struggling into the future. There are actions that we can take to break that cycle of emotional dysregulation, internalized shame, and relationship difficulty and evolve into a new way of living. I have done it, other people have done it, and so can you.

It is very easy to get stuck in a self-defeating mindset where we feel like all of the bad things that we experience from our emotional trauma are an inescapable part of "who we are." While we may be willing to take action and very much want to experience a better quality of life, what may feel real to us is that our life has always been bad, always will be bad, and the only thing we can look forward to is spending the rest of our lives feeling like crap. I call this the "illusion of false fate." False fate is a nagging internal voice that tries to convince us that things will never change, we will never escape from our emotional pain, and that we will always feel stressed, worthless, helpless, or struggle with relationships for the rest of our lives. But that is a lie that emerges from our emotional trauma and only serves to keep us stuck. That sense of helplessness and despair can feel so real and true, but it is not.

I am here to tell you that your past does not have to equal the future. If you are sick of feeling bad about yourself, then you are faced with a choice. While you cannot control how you feel, you do have control over what you do. If you are willing to take the right action, you can evolve into the person you want to become. You are not condemned to being stuck in your past experience, even though it may feel that way sometimes. Open yourself up to the possibility of something different, and make the commitment to take the next little step forward. If you do that every day, even imperfectly, that illusion of false fate will start to fade, and you will start to experience growth toward a healthier and happier future.

3. It Will Become Who You Are

Changing our experience in life requires us to think and act in ways that are different from our normal pattern. While this idea may seem obvious, actually making those changes can be a challenge. When we start setting boundaries, communicating differently, and changing the way we talk to ourselves, there may be a part of us that feels like a fraud, like we are doing something wrong, or that everyone can tell that we are a fake. Stepping out into new territory can feel scary and disorienting. Not only does it require us to act in ways that are unfamiliar, but showing up consistently, authentically, and emotionally engaged in our lives leaves many of us feeling vulnerable and scared. Although we may feel like a fake or like it is "not who we are" when we start making positive changes, it will begin to feel normal to us over time.

There is a part of our brain whose job it is to rationalize and normalize everything that we do, and to cause us to feel anxiety whenever we act differently. Every time we do something, this part of our brain rationalizes our behavior as "just what we do"—even when that behavior is not healthy. This is how people can rationalize their behavior when stealing, drinking themselves into a blackout, or engaging in abusive behavior. Even though they may understand at some level that what they are doing is not right, there is another part of themselves that normalizes their decisions and makes their harmful behavior feel like it is just part of who they are and will come up with all sorts of reasons why it is okay for them to act that way. For those of us with emotional trauma, this rationalizing part of our brain will justify why we push people away, get into fights, struggle to trust, go emotionally numb, blame others, act out in anger, or just about any flavor of destructive behavior.

The rationalizing part of the brain is what we are fighting when we try to make positive changes in our lives. Our old way of thinking, feeling, and acting will feel normal, even though it makes us unhappy. But every time we make a change and do the next right thing for ourselves, even if it makes us uncomfortable, that rationalizing part of the brain will start to normalize it. Over time, what used to make us feel like a fake will feel normal to us. In fact, you should embrace that feeling of being a fake, awkward, or like everyone can tell that you are being a phony when making a positive change. It tells you that what you are doing is breaking out of your old pattern and making progress in your recovery.

4. Focus on Persistence, Not Perfection

Success in your journey does not depend on you being perfect. Just persistent. None of us starts out doing anything perfectly in the beginning. We don't start out by doing math perfectly, swimming perfectly, or navigating through relationships perfectly. In fact, we tend to be pretty lousy at most things in the beginning. The reasons are that learning any new skill takes time, and that development only happens through repetition. While we will often give ourselves plenty of grace when we are fumbling our way through developing any other skill, we often tend to be less forgiving of ourselves when it comes to our own emotional recovery. We tend to want everything immediately, and we become frustrated when we take a step backward or perceive a lack of progress.

I have seen a lot of people transform their lives as well as a lot of people who decide to change, but never seem to make any progress. The difference between them is not how smart they are, how talented they are, how much they know, or even how many therapy sessions they sit through. What separates those who emerge from their emotional trauma to have a happy and meaningful life from those who don't is one simple thing: persistent intentional action. Every time you show up and do the work to make a better life, your mind and soul will shift a little bit in the positive direction. As the famous actor Woody Allen once said, "eighty percent of life is just showing up." If you just keep showing up and doing the work to heal, one day you will look back and realize how much you have evolved. The small things you do imperfectly on a daily basis are far more important than the big things you do perfectly every once in a while. Perfection is much less important than persistence. No matter how imperfect you are, just don't give up.

5. Be Radically Nonjudgmental of Yourself

A challenge for many people with emotional trauma is dealing with the constant mental chatter of negative self-talk that comes from our damaged self-concept. It's like there is some voice in our head that is constantly judging ourselves and the world around us and telling us how much we suck, how much our life sucks, and how much everyone else sucks, too. We will seem to have a genius for interpreting social cues and events in our lives in the most negative way possible, using that as ammunition to further emotionally flagellate ourselves for our perceived flaws, and then becoming angry and resentful. Even when we are able to ignore those voices for a time, there will be moments when all of that negative self-talk comes flooding back in, and we become swept up in a deluge of self-hate or rage toward the world. Getting to a place where we can just see this as a part of our emotional trauma and not judge ourselves can be quite freeing.

When you have emotional trauma, your brain will lie to you a lot. It is just part of the deal. It will try to convince you that you are a flawed and unlovable person, the world is against you, you cannot trust anyone, and you will always be alone. It does this by presenting you with a barrage of evidence that all points to an obvious conclusion: there is something wrong with you and the world is terrible. As long as we listen to what that trauma voice says about us, we will remain trapped in a cycle of self-hate and self-sabotage. However, if we can find a way to see that this negative self-talk is merely a symptom of our wounded self-concept and has nothing to do with reality, then we can start to change our relationship to our inner trauma voice. I have found that an effective way to do this is to adopt a policy of being radically nonjudgmental of yourself.

Self-judgment impairs our ability to see ourselves and our world accurately. Removing that self-judgment helps us have a more accurate view of self and will turn down our criticism of others. An important step toward becoming nonjudgmental is to understand that you have trauma voices in your head that tell you things that aren't true and to decide that you won't base your opinion of yourself and others on what those trauma voices are telling you. It will be important to develop the ability to recognize and accept that you are a wounded and imperfect human being without interpreting this as evidence that there is something wrong with you. You are still a completely lovable human who is worthy of other people's time and attention. You have an inherent right to be treated with dignity and respect, and those who cannot treat you that way are probably the very people who have kept you grounded in your emotional trauma. The goal of being radically nonjudgmental is not to pretend that we are super awesome, it is just to see ourselves accurately.

6. Don't Believe Everything You Think

Truth is what we make when we merge facts about the world with our beliefs about the world. Trauma distorts our sense of what is real and creates a mythology about ourselves and our world that is inaccurate, and then we tend to react emotionally to those myths as though they were real. This happens when we grow up with caregivers who don't have a good grip on reality themselves. Our childhood ends up being one long gaslighting experience. We accepted whatever our parents' version of reality was and learned to distrust our own innate intuition.

We all have adopted a set of beliefs that organize our objective reality into a sense of truth. If those beliefs arise from a damaged self-concept, then the truth we create may not reflect an objective reality at all. For example, when our childhood experience has led us to believe that we are unlovable and worthless, we will merge this belief with our experience to create a truth about ourselves as unlovable. We will tend to perceive facts and events as further proof of our truth. If we adopted the belief that people are dangerous, then we will struggle with a fear of people. If we adopted the belief that we can never do anything right, then we will organize our experiences to make that our truth.

None of this happens intentionally. Our construction of truth from merging our beliefs with the facts happens in the emotional centers of the brain. The emotional part of our brain creates a felt sense of what is true, and the rational part of our brain looks for whatever evidence it can find to support it. Because of this, we have to remember that what feels true may not *be* true. We cannot believe everything we think or everything we feel. If we can open ourselves up to the idea that what feels real to us may not accurately reflect reality, and rely on the perceptions of others whom we trust, we can begin to recalibrate our sense of what is true in a way that helps us see ourselves and the world more accurately.

7. We Cannot Heal on Our Own

As much as it would be nice to be able to read a few books on emotional trauma and then use that information to heal ourselves on our own, that is just not how it works. While doing things like journaling, saying affirmations, and learning about how emotional trauma affects us can be helpful, these techniques alone are not sufficient to create the level of change that will allow us to free ourselves from emotional trauma. We need other people to help us heal.

Not only does surrounding ourselves with safe and sane people model what "normal" looks like, but it also allows others to mirror back to us a more accurate view of ourselves—one that we may not have received growing up. Positive messages from other people affect us at a deeper level than messages we tell ourselves. While saying nice things to ourselves in the mirror feels good in the moment, hearing those same words from others sticks with us and shifts our self-perception in a much more powerful way. Additionally, being able to rely on how other people perceive us gives us a way to check whether our perceptions are accurate or being clouded by our trauma.

Being in an intimate attachment relationship with a healthy partner also helps calm the emotional circuits in our brain and helps us feel safe, loved, connected, empowered, and validated. Emotional attachment bonds that may have been the source of our injury during childhood can become a force for healing as adults.

8. Externalize Your Shame

Internalized shame is a big issue for many of us who have experienced emotional trauma. When we grow up in an environment where the adults in our lives are unable to take accountability for their own behavior, we begin to internalize the sense that we are somehow to blame. Because kids naturally idolize their parents and family, there is a natural tendency to perceive that there is something wrong with us when our parents ignore us, say terrible things to us, make us feel bad about ourselves, or abuse us. We then carry this internalized shame into adulthood in the form of negative self-talk, low self-esteem, and the feeling that we are flawed, wrong, or unlovable.

An important step in our recovery is to turn that internalized shame outward and place it onto the people whose unhealthy behavior undermined the healthy development of our self-concept. It matters little whether their behavior toward us was intentionally harmful or not. We are the ones who end up living with the emotional consequences of inadequate nurturing as children through no fault of our own. Carrying the emotional burden for the adults who were unwilling or incapable of being there for us is not healthy.

Externalizing our shame is recognizing that all that negativity that we carry about ourselves is simply not about us. We are just as lovable and capable as anyone else. The reason we feel that way is that the adults in our lives were not emotionally healthy themselves. It is important to transfer the accountability of how we feel where it belongs. During that process, we may feel angry, resentful, blaming, and all the other intense emotions that come from feeling hurt and somewhat betrayed. We may go through a grieving process about the family that we wished we could have had or for all the time we lost and opportunities we missed because of our emotional trauma. Before we can move onto forgiveness so that we can heal, we have to allow ourselves to feel whatever emotions come up and give them a voice.

9. Forgiving Those Who Hurt You

Resentment toward our parents, partners, or other people who have wounded us is a natural response. After all, we are the ones who are carrying the burden of their behavior toward us, right? It is because of them that we have suffered from the effects of emotional trauma, and now we have to put in all this work in order to heal. We didn't ask for any of this, nor did we deserve it. But now we are facing a lifetime of struggle through no fault of our own, and they get away without any accountability. Anyone who is honest with themselves has had thoughts like this. It is completely normal. What happened to you and me was through no fault of our own, and it was entirely unfair. There is a certain comfort in hanging on to some anger about the whole situation, but if we want to move forward in our recovery, we have to let go of those resentments.

Here is the thing: the anger and resentment that you carry toward those who hurt you does one thing and one thing only. It keeps you emotionally tied to the people and situations that harmed you. Your anger and resentment doesn't help you heal. It doesn't make the people who hurt you feel bad about themselves. It doesn't lead to any resolution. The resentment only keeps you stuck in the role of victim and over time corrodes your soul. But how do you let go of those feelings?

If you want to free yourself from resentments stemming from your past trauma, you need to practice radical forgiveness. Forgiving the people who hurt you for being imperfect human beings does not let them off the hook in some way. It lets you off the hook, emotionally, energetically, and mentally. Forgiveness is more than just intellectually thinking to yourself "they did the best they could," although that is part of it. Forgiveness is projecting compassion toward them for being flawed human beings. It is stepping out of their world, visualizing them as wounded souls, and finding a way to feel sadness for them.

I get how hard this is. I really do. Holding onto hatred for those who hurt us is a much more natural response. Unfortunately, holding onto hatred is one reason it is so difficult to recover from emotional trauma. There is a real tendency to hang onto an emotional thread that keeps us emotionally connected to the very people who hurt us and a part of us tethered to our past. Forgiveness allows us to release our hold on that thread so we can move forward with our life in a positive way.

10. Give Yourself Permission to Evolve

The last principle that I would like to share is to give yourself permission to evolve. Your journey of recovery is much like boarding a ship to sail across the ocean. In the beginning, you may have an idea of where you want to go and even have a general direction to guide you. But you will not be able to see your ultimate destination from the shore from which you embark. That will only be revealed to you as your journey unfolds. The life you visualize for yourself when you start out on your journey of recovery may end up looking different as you begin to heal. That is completely okay. Give yourself permission to evolve. Your only goal should be to keep moving in the right direction and allow the life that is meant for you to be revealed.

As you grow, what feels important to you may evolve as well. That is expected and totally okay. The key is to focus on what is the most important for you at each point in your healing, and pay attention to that. You don't need to apologize or make excuses for why you need to step away from certain acquaintances, relationships, or situations that are keeping you stuck. There are people who would love to know you, support you, and cheer on your success.

Moving Forward

In the next three chapters, we will discuss many tools that can help you on your journey. You will learn strategies to help calm your emotions, heal your core self-concept, and strengthen your relationships. Some of these tools may be more helpful than others, depending on your personal situation and history. That's totally okay. I should also note that there are many more therapies and techniques that are not mentioned in this book. There are just too many options to name them all. Instead, I focused my attention on those that seem to have the longest track record of providing the most benefit.

In the last chapter, we will discuss how to create a holistic and comprehensive plan of action that can help guide you along your journey of recovery. You will learn a simple way to identify where emotional trauma may be impacting you the most so that you can prioritize your time, focus, and energy for maximum benefit. Although this may feel like a lot, just remember that recovery is a process, not a destination, and what may be your biggest challenge today may not be as much of an issue tomorrow. Just relax, cut yourself some slack, and enjoy the journey.

CHAPTER 7

Calming Your Emotions

As we have discussed in previous chapters, emotional dysregulation is one of the hallmarks of emotional trauma. Experiences where we felt trapped and threatened resulted in our limbic system becoming stuck in a state of alarm. Because of this, we will often struggle with emotions that feel intense and unpredictable, will experience intrusive thoughts and emotions from unprocessed memories, and may avoid people or certain situations in an effort to feel safe. We may feel dissociated from our body and emotions, yet have times when we feel flooded with rage, panic, or an ill-defined urgency to escape.

A critical part of our healing journey is to find ways to shift our limbic system out of the alarm response so we can feel more emotionally grounded and calm, and engage in our lives in a more intentional, meaningful, and authentic way. Emotional regulation is the foundation of our recovery from trauma and is important so that we can heal our core self-concept and deepen our relationships with others.

In this chapter, we will talk about four key areas of healing that will help us become more emotionally regulated:

1. Creating a sense of safety
2. Rebuilding our sense of agency
3. Processing trauma memories
4. Making lifestyle changes

Each of these is important. Unless we can create a sense of safety and agency for ourselves, and process our trauma memories, it will be very difficult to shift our limbic system out of a state of alarm and move forward in our recovery. Let's take a look at each of these areas and the specific steps you can take to calm your emotions.

Creating a Sense of Safety

The need for a sense of safety is the most primal of all of our core needs. One of the effects of trauma is for our limbic system to be stuck in a state of alarm, behaving as though we are in danger when we are actually safe. So, we need some tools that will help shift our limbic system out of the alarm response and into a state of calm. Some tools that many of us have found helpful include grounding, rhythmic breathing, trauma-sensitive yoga, creating physical safe spaces, and establishing a support system. Let's take a look at each of these.

Grounding

Grounding is the practice of using our body to communicate to the limbic system that we are safe, thereby reducing our distress and shifting our brain out of the alarm response. This works because of the two-way communication between our body and the limbic system. Not only does the limbic system send messages to our body, but the body also sends messages to our limbic system. By creating a state of calm in our physical body, we can also start to create a state of calm in our brain.

Grounding exercises give us a sense of being present in our body, having awareness of our present-moment experience, feeling our emotions, and reminding ourselves that we are safe. They are simple practices that we can do anywhere whenever we feel ourselves becoming distressed. It is best to begin doing these exercises in a place were we feel safe and won't be disturbed. Over time, it will become easier to do these in other situations.

The Five Senses Exercise

One of the effects of emotional trauma is for us to lose touch with what is happening in the present moment. When trauma memories become triggered, there is a part of us that reexperiences past events as though they are happening now. The Five Senses Exercise helps us turn down the intensity of our distress and reorient ourselves to the present moment.

Here are the steps for this exercise:

1. Start by sitting comfortably with both feet on the floor and your hands resting gently in your lap.

2. Breathe in a slow deep breath and then let it out slowly.

3. Take a look around you and name five things out loud that you can see. For example, "I see a mirror, I see a window, I see the carpet," and so on.

4. Next, direct your attention to four things that you can feel and say them out loud. Feel free to reach out to touch things around you. For example, "I feel my shoes on my feet, I can feel the texture of my pants, I can feel the pressure of the chair against my back," and so on.

5. Next, direct your attention to three things that you can hear and say them out loud. For example, "I can hear the traffic outside, I can hear the fan in the other room, I can hear the chirping of birds."

6. Next, direct your attention to two things you can smell. This may be a challenge because we often block out smells, and you may have to move around a bit to smell different things. For example, "I can smell the flowers on the coffee table, I can smell my sweater," etc. If you can't smell anything, that's okay. Just notice that, and name two of your favorite smells.

7. Last, direct your attention to something that you can taste. The taste in our mouth is also something that we tend to tune out, so you may not be able to name anything unless you have just eaten a mint, had a sip of tea, or recently brushed your teeth. If you can't taste anything in particular, that's okay. Just notice that, and name one of your favorite flavors.

8. Now, take another deep breath in, and slowly let it out.

Once you have finished, take a moment to notice what your body feels like. Do you notice any difference? If so, how would you describe what changed?

Don't be discouraged if it's hard to notice anything different at first. One of the effects of trauma is to dissociate from the sensations in the body, but if you practice this a couple of times per day, it will help you become more grounded in your senses.

Rhythmic Breathing Exercises

When the alert circuit in the limbic system becomes activated, our breathing becomes short and shallow. By intentionally slow-ing down our breathing and breathing deeper, we can communicate to our limbic system that we are safe and it can relax.

Rhythmic breathing is a very simple exercise that you can do anywhere and only requires a few minutes. Intentional and controlled deep breathing helps shift the brain out of the fight-or-flight response and activates the parasympathetic nervous system. Let's take a look at a couple of easy rhythmic breathing exercises that you can start today.

Square Breathing

1. Set a timer for five minutes. Lie down or sit in a comfortable position, close your eyes, and relax.

2. Bring your attention to your breathing. Take a few slow breaths and just pay attention to the sensation of your chest rising as air fills your lungs, and the sensation of your chest dropping as air exits again.

3. When you are ready to begin, count to four as you breathe in, hold your breath for four seconds, slowly release your breath for four seconds, and then hold for four seconds.

That's it. That's the pattern. Four seconds in. Hold for four seconds. Four seconds out. Hold for four seconds. Repeat. The key for this exercise is to focus on the physical sensations in your body as you breathe. When you breathe in, really try to fill your lungs as much as you can. When you breathe out, try to push every last bit of air out to completely empty your lungs.

If you do this exercise every day, you should start noticing a difference in your overall stress level after about two weeks. Some people experience a change right away, but for most people, it takes time. Many people find it beneficial to do this exercise right before bed as it helps improve their sleep.

4-7-8 Breathing

This exercise is essentially the same as the square breathing exercise, but has a different pattern. This pattern is slightly more challenging and may be a bit of a stretch for some people who are just starting.

1. Set a timer for five minutes. Lie down or sit in a comfortable position, close your eyes, and relax.

2. Again, bring your attention to your breathing. Take a few slow breaths and just pay attention to the sensation of your chest rising as air fills your lungs, and the sensation of your chest dropping as air exits again.

3. When you are ready to begin, count to four as you breathe in, hold your breath for seven seconds, slowly release your breath for eight seconds, and then immediately breathe in again.

That's it. That's the pattern. Four seconds in. Hold for seven seconds. Eight seconds out. Repeat. When you breathe in, really try to fill your lungs as much as you can. When you breathe out, try to push every last bit of air out to completely empty your lungs. Like with the square breathing exercise, the key is to focus on the physical sensation of air filling your lungs and then emptying again.

Which one you choose to do is entirely up to you. If you have never done a breathing exercise before, square breathing may be the best place to start. Ultimately, it doesn't matter all that much how many seconds you inhale, hold, or exhale. The point is to be intentional, slow, controlled, and comfortable. That's what will create the desired effect. Most people start out doing the breathing exercises for about five minutes, but may increase the time to ten minutes or more as they become more relaxed and comfortable with the exercise.

CALMING YOUR EMOTIONS

Trauma-Sensitive Yoga

Trauma often leaves us with a sense of disconnection from ourselves, chronic tension in our gut and muscles, and a feeling of being unsafe in our own bodies. Our brain attempts to deal with the constant stress of being stuck in the fight-or-flight response by ignoring the sensations in our body. Unfortunately, by blocking out the feeling of being stressed, we also disconnect from our natural intuition for what is healthy and safe for us, we lose our emotional attunement to other people, and we are deprived of the vibrant sense of being alive. One powerful way that we can calm the nervous system and reconnect with our bodies is through yoga.

Yoga is a practice that combines physical movement with a mindful focus on internal sensations, breathing, and a felt sense of being in the moment. It can be very beneficial for those of us who have experienced emotional trauma because yoga helps us regain a sense of safety, emotional stability, and mental clarity. It helps relax our tense and guarded muscles and restore normal tone to the heart and internal organs.

There is a specific form of yoga called "Trauma-Informed Yoga" or "Trauma-Sensitive Yoga" that is specifically designed to help people with a history of trauma. While it shares most of the same practices as other forms of yoga, Trauma-Sensitive Yoga is much more centered around creating a safe and calm space, using gentle communication, and avoiding poses that can be triggering for some people. Intense emotions and distressing memories can emerge at times during the healing process, and being in a supportive, nonjudgmental environment with a yoga teacher who has experience working with traumatized people is important.

Some of the benefits of Trauma-Sensitive Yoga include:

- More self-compassion and a healthier self-perception
- Feeling more emotionally grounded and calm

- Improved interpersonal relationships
- Improved coping skills to deal with emotional triggers
- Greater sense of cohesion and self-control
- Being better able to stay in the present moment
- Reduced sense of isolation through safe connections with others

Research has shown that yoga is very effective in helping us recover from trauma. Regardless of whether you are a man or a woman, whether your trauma was from childhood or adulthood, yoga is as effective as antianxiety or antidepressant medication in reducing the symptoms of distress, but in a more natural and organic way.

Creating a Physical Safe Space

Part of restoring a sense of safety is to have a physical safe space where you feel calm and secure. A physical safe space is a location where you can retreat whenever you are going through a period when you feel flooded with intense emotion. It can be a room, or even a corner of a room, that is your personal sanctuary to ground and practice self-compassion. Here are a few tips for creating your own safe space:

- Reflect on what makes you feel physically and emotionally safe, and identify some specific boundaries that you want to enforce in your space.
- Communicate what you need from others when you are in your safe space, such as asking before touching you, needing quiet time, or whatever would help you feel comforted.
- Include grounding items like weighted blankets, warm tea, music, daily meditations, nature sounds, or your personal journal.

- If possible, make your space a phone-free, distraction-free, or people-free zone.

Having a physical safe space can be very helpful in our healing journey and is particularly valuable for those of us who grew up in an unsafe environment. The space doesn't have to be big, it just needs to be ours. It should be treated with the same respect as a sanctuary in a house of worship.

Establishing Social Support

Social support is a biological necessity, not an option. We need others to help us regulate our emotions, feel safe, and develop a positive and coherent self-concept. We need the love and support of others to help us restore a sense of safety and agency. This can be hard because many of us with emotional trauma will tend to isolate ourselves out of a fear of being hurt. We may see other people as dangerous and have a hard time with trust, so involving other people in our healing journey may feel scary. However, if we can set aside our fears and engage others, it can help us move forward in a positive way.

Attachment Relationships

As we discussed earlier, emotional attachment bonds to a few close people in our lives is very important for our mental and emotional health. Not only do these attachment relationships help us feel safe, valued, and connected, but they also serve an important role in regulating our emotions. Those close to us can become an emotional shock absorber of sorts, one that serves to tone down the severity of our distress when we are experiencing intense emotions. They can also help us ground and restore a sense of safety by validating our experience, keeping us present, and reassuring us that we are okay.

Ideally, our partner in a committed relationship would be able to provide this for us. But, if we don't have a partner, or our partner is unable to be present with us during times of distress, then close friends, safe family members, clergy, or therapists can provide that kind of support for us. Those of us who experienced attachment trauma growing up may struggle to open up and allow ourselves to be vulnerable to another person. While we need to show ourselves some compassion around how hard it is for us to open up to someone close to us, finding ways to engage our partners, friends, and family will be critical in our healing journey.

Support Groups

Support groups can be very beneficial for those of us who have experienced emotional trauma. They can give us a safe and empathetic space where we can share our experiences, learn coping strategies, and feel less isolated. They can help reduce our sense of isolation, normalize our experiences, and help us feel like we are not alone on our journey of recovery. We may learn practical strategies for managing our symptoms and how to communicate our feelings more effectively.

It's important when we are looking for a support group to find one that feels like a good fit for us. We want a space that feels free of judgment, safe, and organized. If it is facilitated, we want to make sure that the facilitator is trained or has significant practical experience. It is always okay to step back from a group if it feels overwhelming or unhelpful. It doesn't mean that you failed or that you aren't serious about your recovery. Sometimes the people involved in a therapy group just are not a good fit for us for whatever reason. That's okay.

Tapping (Emotional Freedom Technique)

Emotional Freedom Techniques or Tapping, is a form of therapy that uses acupressure points from traditional Chinese medicine in combination with cognitive-behavioral therapy to help reduce emotional distress. The basic concept is that by tapping on specific meridian points on the face and upper body while focusing on a specific feeling, problem, or trauma memory, the energy behind the emotions and memories is reduced and the energy system of the body is rebalanced. Although no one is exactly sure how this works, many people have found tapping to be very helpful. Tapping is not specifically just for trauma. It can be used to help decrease anxiety before giving a presentation, as preparation for a difficult conversation, or anytime when you want to calm yourself. Getting into the details of how to do tapping is beyond the scope of this chapter, but many books and online resources are available to teach you how to do this simple technique.

Rebuilding a Sense of Agency

Our second step is rebuilding a sense of agency. The violation of the need for a sense of agency is the one of the elements of a traumatic experience. It is the feeling of being trapped and helpless that makes an otherwise stressful event into a traumatic one. Rebuilding a sense of agency after trauma means that we are reclaiming our ability to make choices, set boundaries, and be an active agent in our lives who can intentionally direct the way in which we interact with the world. To the extent that we can do this, we shift ourselves away from the sense of victimhood where we feel like life happens to us, to a place of empowerment where we feel that our actions, efforts, and decisions will determine the outcome of our life.

When we have a strong sense of agency, we can acknowledge situations where we have been overpowered and hurt, but those situations do not represent evidence that we are powerless in general. Defensive aggression, avoiding people, people pleasing, and emotional numbing are all common ways that we may try to cope with the a damaged sense of agency. As we become more empowered, these compensatory coping mechanisms will tend to fade, and we will feel less triggered or shut down by setbacks or challenges.

Making Choices

Trauma, by definition, is not something that we can choose. It's the nonconsensual nature of the painful event that makes it emotionally traumatizing. But feeling a lack of agency is not just from experiencing a series of traumatic events. It can also result from growing up in an environment where someone else made all the decisions for us and didn't allow us the room to make decisions for ourselves. When this happens, we may feel very insecure about our own choices and have difficulty voicing our preferences to others. So, one of the steps in creating our internal sense of agency is to make choices and own them. When we make a decision, we are putting a stake in the ground and proclaiming to the world, "This is what I want, and what I am deciding to do."

We can start by making low-stakes choices like what to wear, when to eat, when to exercise, or what you are going to do over the weekend, and then celebrating following through on those choices. As silly as it may sound, simply deciding where to go for lunch and then celebrating your success when you actually go there for lunch can be an important first step. You may find it helpful to start out with a series of wins from making small decisions and following through on them. Every successful choice will have an effect on how you feel about yourself and your ability to affect the world around you.

Setting Boundaries

Boundaries are the internal psychological structure that we create to organize our experiences, define our self-concept, shape our self-perception, and establish the edge between where we end and where the world around us begins. Trauma disrupts the formation of our internal and external boundaries either by disrupting their formation, as in the case of attachment trauma, or by violating them through force, as in the case of acute trauma. In either case, the internalized helplessness and vulnerability that often results from the struggle to set and maintain healthy boundaries can keep our brain stuck in the alarm response.

An important step in your recovery from emotional trauma is to learn how to set and maintain healthy boundaries, both when it comes to our self-concept (internal boundaries) and how we allow others to interact with us (external boundaries). While most of us know the importance of setting healthy boundaries, we may find it very difficult to achieve. One of the challenges is that many of us don't really have a good sense of what healthy boundaries even look like. If we grew up in a chaotic or dysfunctional home where our parents or caregivers did not have healthy boundaries, trying to set healthy boundaries can feel like we are having to re-create a painting that we have never seen.

Another challenge for many of us is that our previous attempts at setting boundaries for ourselves were often met with aggression, shaming, or some form of retribution. This is particularly true if we had parents or partners who were narcissistic, had an addiction, or were abusive. Because of this, the idea of setting and holding healthy boundaries may feel quite terrifying at some level. Even asking someone to stop talking to you in a disrespectful way can feel scary.

If setting healthy boundaries has been a challenge for you, here are a few things that may help:

- Start small. Experiencing success setting small boundaries will help you be more successful in setting bigger ones. This may be as simple as setting aside a period of time each day that is just for you, or deciding to pursue a hobby that is simply for your enjoyment, and making the decision that you will not feel guilty for it.

- Notice patterns in your life that tend to create distress. Do you take on too much at work? Do you have trouble saying no? Do you find yourself always accommodating the needs of others to your own detriment? Make a list of those things, and then write down some ideas about how you could show up in a healthier way in those situations. What could you say differently? How could you hold a boundary for yourself?

- Break the habit of feeling like you have to justify yourself when setting a boundary. Just practice saying "no", or "I am not comfortable talking about that with you", or "I am sorry, but I need some time for myself this weekend", and then stopping. This can feel very hard when we are used to putting everyone else's needs first. Just remind yourself that you are not being selfish. You are showing up in your life in a healthier way.

Journaling to Build Agency

Journaling can be a very helpful form of therapy to help reduce internalized shame, build a sense of agency, integrate our experiences into a larger narrative of our life, and find some meaning in our experience. It provides a safe, private space for us to process our experiences when talking about them causes us to become flooded with distress. It allows us to slow everything down and get our feelings out of our head and onto the page where we can see them more clearly. Because we can choose when we write, what we write, and what we focus on, journaling can help us create a sense of agency over our experience. If we journal on a regular basis, it also allows us to see our growth over time and how we have evolved.

Journaling can focus on different things, depending on what feels helpful to us in the moment. Here are a few ways that you could use journaling in your healing journey:

- **Expressive writing.** Write your thoughts and feelings in the moment for a set amount of time without any regard to organization. This could be for five minutes, fifteen minutes, or whatever feels comfortable.

- **Narrative journaling.** Write your life story from when you were a child to where you are today, highlighting all of the significant events, both good and bad. The intent is to create a continuous narrative of our lives to help place our trauma as an event in our past.

- **Dialoguing.** Write out a conversation with your inner child, the trauma, or other people in your life. What would you say to your younger self? If you could speak to the part of you that holds your trauma, what would it want to hear from you?

- **Gratitude journaling.** Write about what you are grateful for to help restore a sense of hope, connection, or self-compassion. If you struggle to find gratitude, what would you like to feel grateful for?

- **Body-based journaling.** Write about the physical sensations in your body and what they might be expressing emotionally. This is very helpful in helping us create the connection between our mind and body.

Any time we are addressing the emotions associated with our trauma, we want to do so in a way that allows us to be present without getting triggered. Here are a few tips for ensuring that your journaling is a healing experience for you:

- Go slowly—you don't have to revisit the most painful parts right away.

- Ground yourself afterward—deep breaths, gentle movement, or a comforting routine.
- Don't force insight—sometimes just writing is enough.
- Have support available, especially if intense feelings arise.
- Give yourself permission to vary the types of journaling you do; one day you may focus on gratitude journaling, the next day you might choose to do narrative journaling.

Writing about our experience and emotional struggles can be a very powerful form of therapy. It was certainly a powerful tool in my own recovery.

Processing Trauma Memories

Our third step in calming our emotions is processing our trauma memories. As we discussed earlier, the way in which trauma memories are stored in the brain is one of the main reasons why we become stuck in the fight-or-flight response, even though the danger has passed. Whereas nontraumatic events are encoded into long-term memory as coherent narratives about past experiences, traumatic events are not encoded in the same way. They continue to be pulled into the present moment and our emotions respond as though there is a part of us that is still living in that frightening place. So, an important part of calming our emotions is to find ways to process those trauma memories out of the present and into our long-term memory as events that happened in our past. Here are a few healing therapies that have been helpful for many people.

Art Therapy

Art therapy has the ability to bypass the limitations of language and tap into the nonverbal realm of human experience where trauma often resides. You might not always describe your feelings accurately, especially if your trauma involves memory gaps or physical sensations you can't fully articulate. The creative process activates several regions of your brain simultaneously, including areas associated with sensory processing, emotional regulation, and memory encoding. It helps us express, process, and integrate our experiences in a way that talk therapy cannot. Art therapy offers several benefits compared to other forms of trauma therapy:

1. **Engages nonverbal expression.** Trauma is often stored in parts of the brain that don't process language easily. Art allows access to those feelings and memories without needing to talk about them.

2. **Restores control.** Creating art lets you make choices—color, shape, size, subject—rebuilding agency and a sense of safety.

3. **Regulates emotions.** The process of making art can calm the nervous system, reduce anxiety, and create space for reflection.

4. **Rewires the brain.** Engaging in creative expression can help integrate traumatic memories into your broader life story.

If you want to do some art therapy on your own, here are a few ideas you could try:

- Create a drawing or painting of your feelings. This helps to externalize our emotions and gives them a sense of form. After creating a painting of your current emotional experience, you may want to create another drawing or painting of what a healthy form of that same emotion may look like.

- Create a "trauma timeline" or life timeline that marks the significant events in your life, both positive and negative.

You can use different colors or symbols to represent different types of events, such as traumatic experiences, happy memories, and turning points. This helps to place the trauma within the larger context of your life as an event that happened to you in your past, rather than something that is happening to you currently.

- Create a self-portrait or mask of yourself that represents how you see yourself, both physically and emotionally. This may help reveal some inner thoughts about yourself that would have been difficult to put into words. You can use colors, symbols, or words to express different aspects of your identity. You could also create a self-portrait that is a vision for your future or a self-portrait of what your healed self would be like.

- Create a drawing or painting of a place where you feel safe, calm, and at peace. It can be a real place or an imaginary one. Focus on the atmosphere, colors, or shapes that foster safety for you. Concentrate on how you feel as you create.

- Create a drawing or painting that outlines your body. Inside the outline, draw or write about the physical sensations and emotions you experience in different parts of your body when thinking about the traumatic event. This exercise helps you to identify where you sense emotional distress or relief in your own body.

There are many different ways that art can be implemented into your healing journey. We have touched on only a few of them here. You may find that the creative artistic process opens up avenues of expression and emotional processing that feel deeper and more complete than trying to express those same experiences through language.

CALMING YOUR EMOTIONS

Eye Movement Desensitization and Reprocessing (EMDR)

A therapy called "eye movement desensitization and reprocessing" (EMDR) can be very helpful in shifting the brain out of the fight-or-flight response and is a very effectie treatment for emotional trauma. It was discovered by accident in 1987 by the psychologist Francine Shapiro as she was walking through a park one day trying to avoid working on her dissertation. As she walked along preoccupied with some painful memories, she noticed that some of the disturbing thoughts that she was having were suddenly disappearing. When she recalled them again, she was surprised that they weren't as distressing as they had been only a few minutes prior. Curiously, when she brought up another painful memory, she noticed that her eyes started darting back and forth in a particular way. What Dr. Shapiro had stumbled upon was a fascinating clue about the way in which the brain uses bilateral movement and stimulation to process and encode memory.

It turns out that a traumatized brain has difficulty processing and storing memories associated with its own trauma. So rather than the memories of those events being stored properly and recalled as bad things that happened in the past, they are stuck in the present and continuously reexperienced as though they are happening in the here and now. Instead of being able to emotionally distance ourselves from traumatic events through time and distance, as we can with normal memories about a previous time in a different place, we can only escape from the terror of what is happening in the present moment through dissociation. Revisiting traumatic experiences can be detrimental if those memories are still stuck in the present and only being kept at bay through dissociation. Trying to dig into your past to reconnect with traumatic experiences while they are still in the present is often retraumatizing because you are essentially punching holes in the only barrier that is keeping your brain from flooding with distress. At the same time, living with the dissociation, agitation, and flashbacks from unprocessed trauma isn't the answer either.

EMDR is a specific technique that utilizes forms of bilateral physical stimulation or movement along with guided visualization to reprocess traumatic events out of our present experience and into stored memory. This provides us with a sense of separation between what happened in the past and what is happening right now. EMDR allows us to put trauma in its rightful place as past experiences, and decouples those memories from our fight-or-flight response. When EMDR works, we may still feel sadness, anger, or fear from recalling those memories, but the intrusiveness and the uncontrolled flooding of distress should be gone, or at least dramatically reduced.

Interestingly, while EMDR is the gold-standard treatment for adult-onset PTSD from a single event or period of time, it is much less effective as a stand-alone therapy for people with a history of attachment trauma. A 2007 study by Bessel van der Kolk showed that those who had experienced trauma as adults had a 73% cure rate with EMDR eight months after the end of therapy, compared to 25% who had experienced attachment trauma while growing up. In reflecting on the findings van der Kolk states:

> Chronic childhood abuse causes very different mental and biological adaptations than discrete traumatic events in adulthood. EMDR is a powerful treatment for stuck traumatic memories, but it doesn't necessarily resolve the effects of the betrayal and abandonment that accompany physical or sexual abuse in childhood.

This makes sense because when trauma happens in adulthood, it typically does not have the impact on the sense of self that a pattern of emotional trauma has on a developing child. The damage to the core self becomes a psychological anchor for the trauma that tends to trap the traumatic memories in the present for as long as the damage to the core self remains. This puts people with emotional trauma in a difficult spot because it implies that we can't get our brain out of the fight-or-flight response until we heal the core self, and we can't heal the core self until we can get our brain out of the fight-or-flight response. This catch-22 is one of the reasons why the effects of childhood trauma can be so difficult to effectively treat. Combining EMDR therapy with healing strategies for the core self seems to be the most effective way of addressing both simultaneously so that progress can occur.

Psychedelic Therapy

Psychedelic therapy for emotional trauma involves using psychedelic substances, such as MDMA, psilocybin, or ketamine, as part of therapy. Although this is still considered somewhat controversial, a number of studies that have shown that the use of psychedelic medications can have a significant benefit for those struggling with the emotional effects of trauma. The way this seems to work is that these psychedelic drugs promote neuroplasticity in the brain, which may help the brain to reprocess traumatic memories more effectively and reduce the intensity of distress and fear, which allows people to confront and process intense emotions and memories without becoming overwhelmed. The studies that have been done on the use of psychedelics so far have been very promising, suggesting that it may provide relief for some people with trauma that doesn't respond to other forms of therapy. If you are going to try psychedelic therapy as part of your healing journey, be sure to do it under the direction of a licensed medical professional.

Making Lifestyle Changes

In addition to creating a sense of safety, building a sense of agency, and processing trauma memories, there are some lifestyle changes that we can make as well to help us calm our emotions, including avoiding unhealthy situations and toxic people, minimizing our consumption of alcohol, engaging in vigorous exercise, and minimizing our exposure to the news and social media.

Avoid Unhealthy Situations and Toxic People

It will be much more difficult to shift our brain out of the alarm response if we are in situations where we feel emotionally or physically unsafe, whether it's at work, at home, or in the neighborhood. A tragic tendency for many people who have experienced emotional trauma is to be oddly unwilling to leave toxic relationships or environments. While there are certainly situations where individuals are trapped in unhealthy situations due to a lack of resources, opportunity, or a fear of retribution, there are many who stay even when they have the opportunity to leave.

Oftentimes this arises from a pattern that was established in childhood where we learned to adapt to a dysfunctional family environment that was unsafe and where our own emotional needs were not important. Existing in an unhealthy family and social system may feel normal and have a certain familiarity that tends to draw us in. Even though we may hate how we feel, stepping away from jobs, relationships, or peer groups that are are harmful may seem like a bridge that is difficult to cross.

While it is not always easy to get out of unhealthy situations, it will be very difficult to calm our emotions and begin to heal while we are still living in a physical or emotional combat zone. An important step in our healing journey is to recognize unhealthy situations and give ourselves permission to avoid or step away from them. It may be helpful to start out each day by asking yourself three questions:

- What people, relationships, or situations are in my life right now that make me feel unsafe to show up as my authentic self?

- What are some ways that I can disconnect from unhealthy people and environments and engage with those where I feel loved and supported?

- What step can I take today to put myself in a healthier situation where I feel safe and empowered?

We may have a hard time extracting ourselves from unhealthy situations out of a misplaced sense of duty or responsibility for the happiness and well-being of others. We may feel like we want to save them from having to experience pain and may feel like we are letting them down if we walk away. Feelings like this arise from our wounded sense of self and will keep us stuck. Even though it may feel awkward, being very intentional about avoiding unhealthy people and situations will help us create a sense of safety.

Minimize Your Consumption of Alcohol

While in small quantities, alcohol can help calm the nervous system, it also has the effect of dysregulating our emotions or allowing us to numb ourselves. Over time, alcohol use may make our symptoms worse. Here's why:

- Alcohol is a depressant, which can intensify feelings of sadness, hopelessness, or anxiety. There can also be a rebound effect where we feel emotionally worse once the effect wears off.

- Those of us with emotional trauma may already have disrupted sleep, and while alcohol may help us fall asleep initially, it tends to disrupt the restorative REM sleep that is important for our mental health.

- Alcohol impairs our ability to regulate our emotions, which can lead to emotional outbursts and changes in personality that are unhealthy both for us and for those around us.

- Those of us with emotional trauma are at a high risk of abusing alcohol or other substances as a way to suppress our intrusive thoughts and suppress our emotional pain. Although it may help us cope with those feelings in the moment, the dysregulating effects of alcohol will often make our symptoms worse over time.

The bottom line here is that it may be best to avoid alcohol consumption until you have had the opportunity to heal and your emotional system is well-regulated. If you choose to consume alcohol, really try to limit your intake.

Minimize Social Media and the News

Some elements of the modern news and social media environment are essentially a pipeline of highly concentrated emotional sewage intended to induce a sense of shock and impotent outrage in those who consume it. This wasn't always the case, but as the social and political climate has become more toxic and less constrained by social decency, so have the news and social media. Doom scrolling on social media can be addictive for sure, but it is not helpful for those of us with emotional trauma because it tends to trigger the alert circuit in the brain and increase our level of stress.

You may benefit from cutting out media completely. It's not like the universe will stop revolving or you will miss out on something important if you tune out. If anything, as your attention shifts away from an artificially constructed reality toward an organic one, you will likely find new ways to become engaged in activities that feed your soul and calm your mind.

Moving Forward

One of the goals in our recovery from emotional trauma is to calm our emotions so that we are not constantly stuck in a state of tension. We can do this by creating a sense of safety, establishing a sense of agency, processing trauma memories into long-term memory, and making some lifestyle changes. The techniques for calming our emotons that we talked about in this chapter are not the only ways to do so. You may have tried other therapies or techniques that have been helpful. Regardless of how we get there, our goal is simple: to get our brain to relax so we can heal.

This part of your journey will take some time. Give yourself permission to work at a pace that is sustainable and be compassionate toward yourself. If you make your healing a part of your everyday life, rather than a goal to be achieved, it will be easier to stick with it. Slow and methodical will get you to your goal faster than trying to do everything at once.

CHAPTER 8

Healing Your Core Self-Concept

EARLIER IN THE BOOK, we discussed the idea of the core self-concept as a deep psychological structure that shapes our experience of life by organizing the way in which we perceive ourselves and our world. It is highly attuned to interpret social and environmental cues around five existential needs that are critical for our well-being: a sense of identity, a sense of connection, a sense of safety, a sense of value, and a sense of agency. Our experience with our parents and other caregivers during childhood either facilitated or disrupted the development of how we perceive ourselves around these five needs.

If we grew up in a stable and safe home with loving and responsive parents, these five areas of our self-concept likely developed in a healthy way and provided us with a general feeling of being safe, lovable, empowered, and emotionally bonded to our family, and with a good sense of who we are. However, if we grew up in homes that were marked by violence, uninvolved parents, or caregivers, an unstable or chaotic living situation, or caregivers who shamed or mocked us, some of these critical needs would not have been met, and parts of our self-concept would not have developed properly.

The holes in the structure of our core self-concept that resulted from not getting the emotional nurturing that we needed will tend to impact us in three important ways. First, the lack of development of a part of ourselves will leave us feeling damaged in that area. For example, if our sense of value was not nurtured and didn't develop properly, we will tend to struggle with feelings of being broken, unlovable, unworthy, or unwanted—even when we are loved by the people around us. If our sense of safety did not develop properly, we may struggle with fear, anxiety, and a lack of trust—even when we are not in danger.

Second, the holes in our self-concept will affect how we perceive ourselves and the world around us. For example, if we have a hole in our sense of value, we will tend to perceive events in our life as further evidence of how worthless we are. If we have a hole in our sense of safety, we will tend to perceive the events in our life as further evidence of how dangerous people are or how they can't be trusted. If we have a hole in our sense of agency, we will tend to perceive ourselves as helpless to affect the events in our lives or have difficulty setting boundaries.

Third, we will seek to fill the hole in our sense of self by trying to satisfy that particular need, but we usually do this in an unhealthy way. For example, if our sense of value was not nurtured, we may engage in people-pleasing behaviors in an unconscious attempt to get people to recognize our value. If our sense of safety was not nurtured, we may seek safety through avoiding people, or engage in fawning behavior toward an unsafe partner.

Part of our journey of recovery from emotional trauma is to learn how to recognize when these negative feelings, distorted perceptions, and unhealthy behaviors are being activated, and learn new ways to relate to those wounded parts of ourselves. One way that I have found helpful is to give a name to the wounded parts of ourselves that try to make us feel things that aren't true, perceive things that aren't real, and engage in behaviors that undermine our own happiness and success. I call these parts of ourselves our personal demons.

Our Personal Demons

Our personal demons are simply parts of our core self-concept that have been wounded and are using emotional pain to get our attention. They are fed through our distorted perception of ourselves and reinforced by our self-defeating behaviors. Because they emerge from our own woundedness, our personal demons tend to be annoying lifelong partners who actively undermine our quality of life and never seem to go away on their own. Once they start flooding us with emotion, they often take control of our ability to think, feel, and act in a healthy way, and they push us out of the driver's seat of our own lives.

I know that some people may be uncomfortable with the word "demon," but I am not using the term in a biblical sense. Demons are not external evil entities that are trying to corrupt our souls by exploiting our weak points and insecurities. They are simply injured parts of ourselves that are clamoring for our attention because they desperately want to be healed. They just don't know how to ask politely.

Demons Are Lousy Communicators

One thing that is just a truism about personal demons is that they are really bad at communication. They cannot just tap us on the shoulder and say "Excuse me, but I seem to have this poor sense of value here that needs some support. Do you think you can spare a moment to take a look?" Our demons can't do that because the wounds from emotional trauma reside in nonverbal areas of the brain. Oftentimes the only message that we get when one of our demons is triggered is an ill-defined and intense emotional reaction. When there seem to be no words to capture the emotional flooding and internal collapse that we are experiencing, it is a good sign that something has triggered one of our demons, and we are in the middle of a trauma reaction. If we learn some tools to help us recognize and interpret the emotional signals that our wounded parts are sending us, we can gain a new understanding of ourselves and begin healing.

The Five Personal Demons

Since our personal demons emerge from the woundedness to our core self-concept, there are five different ones that can take up residency in our heads, depending on which of our existential needs has not been met. I call these the demons of Disorientation, Isolation, Fear, Unlovability, and Helplessness. Each of them will tend to be triggered by different situations and events, flood us with different emotions, affect how we perceive things differently, and lead to different behaviors. Let's take a quick look at each of these.

The Demon of Disorientation

When the need for a sense of identity is not developed in a healthy way, our Demon of Disorientation will tend to make us feel empty, rudderless, lost, and like we are constantly trying to find ourselves. We will tend to take on the interests and beliefs of those around us to an unhealthy degree and will seem to become a different person in different social situations. We will often struggle with consistency, staying on task, and maintaining focus, and we will tend to act in impulsive and unpredictable ways.

The Demon of Isolation

When the need for a sense of connection is not developed in a healthy way, our Demon of Isolation will tend to make us feel bored, alone, and rejected, or that life is meaningless. We may struggle with resentment and anger from the perceived rejection of others, and we may fantasize about making other people hurt like we do just so we don't feel so alone. We will tend to isolate ourselves when distressed, struggle to maintain friendships and relationships, and may struggle to engage with others when we are with a group of people.

The Demon of Fear

When the need for a sense of safety is not developed in a healthy way, our Demon of Fear will tend to make us feel anxious, distrusting, paranoid, or filled with a sense of dread. We may become convinced that people will end up hurting us if we let our guard down, become suspicious of their motives, and expect disappointment whenever things are going well in our lives. We will tend to be defensive, critical, and guarded toward people, and either act with anger toward others or avoid engaging with them.

The Demon of Unlovability

When the need for a sense of value is not developed in a healthy way, the Demon of Unlovability will tend to make us feel numb, depressed, dirty, broken, or worthless. We may feel like our friendship with someone is a burden on them, and feel that if people really knew who we were, they wouldn't like us. We may struggle to assert ourselves out of the fear that any inconvenience on the other person's part would make them feel like we are not worth the effort. We may push people away when they get too close to us, engage in self-harming behaviors, and struggle to advocate for ourselves.

The Demon of Helplessness

When the need for a sense of agency is not developed in a healthy way, the Demon of Helplessness will tend to make us feel hopeless, incapable, or immobilized. We may feel like no matter what we do, nothing ever works out, that life just happens to us, and that everything is inescapably catastrophic. We may struggle to set boundaries and tend to make everyone else's needs more important than our own. We may seek ways to escape from a life where we feel trapped, overwhelmed, and out of control, and may engage in self-destructive control behaviors such as eating disorders, addictions, or even suicide.

Most of us will have two or three of these demons that are responsible for most of our mental and emotional pain. If you grew up in an extremely toxic environment, you may have damage to all five parts of your core self-concept. However, it is more common to have at least a couple areas that are developed just fine and a couple areas that are not. For example, we may feel very confident in our abilities to accomplish anything, but struggle with the Demons of Unlovability and Isolation. We may feel that we are a very lovable person and have good sense of emotional bond with our loved ones, but struggle with the Demons of Fear, Disorientation, and Helplessness.

Again, you don't necessarily have to call them demons if there is another name that resonates better. But giving those wounded parts of ourselves a name and framing them as independent entities allows us to form a different relationship with them and helps to put us back in the driver's seat of our own lives. Let's take a look at specific steps you can take to build a healing relationship with your personal demons.

In the Moment and Every Day

The work that we will be doing to repair the damage to our core self-concept falls into two basic categories: what to do in the moment when we feel one of our personal demons getting triggered, and work that we can do every day, regardless of whether we feel triggered or not. The "in the moment work" will center around recognizing emotional inflection points that signal to us that one or more of our demons is getting triggered and then using some reparenting skills to help us heal that wounded part of ourselves. The "every day work" will center around maintaining a daily recovery journal where we can develop a new narrative of our life and become more of an active agent in our own healing.

In both the work we do in the moment whenever one of our personal demons gets triggered, and in the work we do every day in our daily recovery journal, we will focus on three things: negative feelings, distorted perceptions, and unhealthy behaviors. These are the three ways that holes in our core self-concept tend to show up, and they are the three areas that we want to track to measure our recovery process over time.

In the Moment: Emotional Inflection Points and Reparenting

We introduced the concept of emotional inflection points in a previous chapter as a moment when there is a sudden shift in emotional tone. In the context of a relationship, inflection points tend to show up during times of relationship distress or conflict, and often mark the point where conflict begins to escalate. In the context of our everyday life, inflection points tend to happen whenever one of our personal demons becomes triggered from some otherwise benign event. They could be triggered by someone looking at us or saying something the wrong way, a social media post, remembering something from our past, or just about anything, really. The important point to remember is that emotional inflection points don't just come out of nowhere, even though it may seem that way. They are triggered for a reason, and that reason is that we are perceiving something that speaks to our wounded core self-concept in some way.

One of the challenges of emotional inflection points is that they happen very fast, and it is not always easy to tell when we are experiencing one. There are times we can go from being calm to becoming flooded with distress or emotionally shutting down in what seems like an instant. So, part of our processing of inflection points is to try to slow everything down and pay attention to the negative feelings that are coming up, what has shifted in how we are perceiving ourselves, and what actions seem urgent to take. Let's take a closer look at each of these components of an inflection point.

Negative Feelings

When one of our demons gets triggered, we will tend to feel a sudden, and often strong, shift in our emotional state. One moment we may feel fine and the next minute, it's like a flood of emotion emerges from our gut. Depending on which of our personal demons gets triggered, we may experience a sense of rage, despair, panic, going numb, or feeling like we are emotionally collapsing on the inside. During these times, this sudden shift in emotion tends to permeate everything, and we will have difficulty experiencing anything other than the flooding emotion.

Distorted Perceptions

Our perceptions of ourselves and the world also become distorted when a demon gets triggered. It is like our brain suddenly sees everything in our life as some kind of evidence for the truth of what we are feeling, and because these distorted perceptions are linked to strong emotions from our damaged sense of self, they will feel deeply true and so obvious to us that we tend to reject anything to the contrary. We may become convinced that our partner is cheating on us, or that someone is trying to hurt us, or that everyone hates us, or that everything we do is a failure, and there is nothing that anyone can say to change our mind. We lose our ability to be flexible in our thinking or to look at things from another perspective. Instead, we become locked into the only reality that feels deeply true to us in the moment.

Unhealthy Behaviors

The intense emotions and distorted perceptions may drive us to act out in sudden, impulsive, and sometimes extreme ways. We may suddenly end relationships, become confrontational, isolate ourselves, get stuck in a storm of rage, jump into our car and drive to nowhere, destroy things that were once meaningful to us, or engage in self-destructive behaviors like cutting, alcohol, drugs, excessive spending, or sexual behaviors that are outside of what is normal for us.

The Inflection Point Exercise

When we experience an emotional inflection point, there is a process that we can follow to help us remain present and in control of our emotions, and begin to heal the wounded parts of ourselves that are causing this to happen. These four steps will help you recognize when one of your demons is being triggered, hold space for your experience without becoming flooded by it, listen to the message your wounded parts are trying to tell you, and then comfort that part of you that is being triggered. Let's take a look at each of these steps and then go through a couple of examples.

Step 1: Identify the Moment of Inflection

The first step is to recognize when one of your demons gets triggered. As soon as you recognize the emotional shift, stop for a moment to experience what is coming up, and then state something out loud like "I can feel myself reacting right now", or perhaps, "Something is coming up for me right now." If you are not in a place where you can say anything out loud, then just say it to yourself silently.

This quick three-part process of recognizing when something gets triggered, pausing for a moment to feel what is coming up, and then calling out your change of emotional state does a couple of important things. First, it slows down your reaction to the emotional inflection point and allows you to remain in control. Second, it changes your relationship to the triggered emotions by externalizing them, which allows us to maintain a better sense of objectivity.

Because these emotional triggers have been part of our lives for so long, we may not immediately recognize when they happen. We may just find ourselves in a triggered state and may not be sure how we ended up there. That's okay. Just do this step whenever you recognize that you are in a triggered state. Over time, you will be better able to recognize emotional inflection points as they happen.

Step 2: Hold Space for the Emotions and Sensations

Once you recognize that a trauma response has been triggered, the next step is to hold space for your experience and allow it to exist somewhere in your body. Many people find it helpful to visualize a spherical space or a bubble inside their gut where the intense emotions can be contained, held, and protected. If you can, give those emotions some form or shape. Are they gray or colorful? Are they amorphous like clouds, or do they have structure? Do they move around inside the bubble or are they stationary? Don't try to force an idea of what they should look like, just observe and notice if there is any form to them at all. If not, that's okay.

If you are able to do this, remember that you are holding a wounded part of yourself that is trying to heal. Show it some compassion and treat it as you would a child who is hurt and frightened. Don't feel bad if you struggle to do this perfectly right away. It takes some practice. Just do the best you can.

Step 3: Ask the Triggered Emotion Why It Is Up Right Now

Now that we have the triggered emotions held safely in our gut, we want to find out what they are trying to tell us. After all, our wounded parts get triggered for a reason. There is something that they are trying to tell us. Look at the bubble that is holding the triggered emotions and ask "Why are you up right now?", or "What are you trying to tell me?"

Pause for a moment to see what messages come up. Are there any images or memories that emerge? Are there any words or phrases that come to mind? Whatever comes up, just notice it and accept it. If nothing comes up, that's fine too. Just notice that without judgment. Our deep emotional wounds, particularly from early childhood, are not always able to communicate with us very well.

Step 4: Reparenting Your Demons

This last step is where we reparent the wounded parts of ourselves that is being triggered. Most of our demons are wounded parts of ourselves that exist because we did not have adequate parenting during childhood. There was something that kept the adults in our lives from being emotionally present in a way to facilitate the healthy development of our core self-concept. The good news is that as adults, we can speak to our wounded parts and give our younger self the care and support that we did not receive during childhood.

If we imagine what an ideal parent would say to us when we were hurt or frightened, and say those things to the triggered emotions we are holding in our gut, we can begin to comfort those wounded parts and help them heal. We may want to say something like, "I know that you feel upset right now, but I am here with you, and you are going to be okay." Or perhaps something like, "It is okay for you to feel afraid. I want you to know that you are going to be fine, and I will protect you from being hurt again." Whatever messaging feels right for you is great, as long as it validates the emotion, comforts the wounded part, and then gives some word of encouragement and support.

Applying These Four Steps

Here is an example of an extreme inflection point that I experienced while I was still in high school. Let's use the steps that we just learned to make sense of what happened to me, and how these four steps could have been used to navigate the situation differently.

"The Most Perfect Family in the World"

Jerry was the most genuinely nice guy that I knew in high school. While almost everyone else in my class treated me with as much kindness as they would a piece of gum stuck to the bottom of their shoe, Jerry would break out in a big smile every time he saw me. He didn't care that my clothes were totally not cool, that my hair wasn't washed, or that I was solidly placed in the "loser" social strata of the school. For some reason, he wanted to be my friend. He often invited me over to his house during lunchtime for sandwiches, we wrote stupid poems and laughed, and we listened to his massive collection of Frank Zappa albums. His father was the same way. Every time his dad saw me, he shook my hand with a big smile on his face and talked to me like I was his own son. To this day, I don't know that I have ever met a more genuinely happy and kind family. That was the problem.

What Jerry and his father didn't see was how dark and empty I was inside. How could they? It was obvious that the bond they shared filled each other's lives with such a sense of happiness that they simply had no frame of reference to comprehend how different my experience was. As they smiled and showered me with kindness, it highlighted how alone and broken I felt. The disparity between their vibrance and my emptiness was often painful to experience.

I ended our friendship shortly after an experience I had at their house one night. Jerry and his father were in the living room, and I was walking back to them after grabbing something to drink in the kitchen. As I entered the doorway, I saw the two of them sitting on the couch next to each other laughing. His dad had his arm over Jerry's shoulders and they both looked at me with big smiles on their faces as they saw me enter. I can still see them sitting there looking at me as though it happened yesterday. So happy. So content. So brimming with love and life. It was just too painful for me to see. I felt my gut drop, a flood of panic swept over my body, and I felt like I was going to physically throw up. I had to get out of there. The urgency to flee suddenly felt so intense that I quickly ran out of their house and into the cold night where the familiar cloak of darkness and isolation could once again envelop and comfort me.

I have thought a lot about that experience over the years. Here was a situation where I was accepted and loved by Jerry and his family, yet I found the experience to be triggering and painful, rather than happy and nurturing. Unfortunately, one of the effects of emotional trauma is that we tend to instinctively recoil from the very people and situations that would be healthy and supportive for us because we don't understand how to navigate through healthy situations, and they tend to heighten our awareness of our own pain. That was certainly the case for me.

Let's walk through this experience to illustrate how I could have navigated this situation differently had I known how to use the four steps we outlined.

1. What was the inflection point?

When I saw Jerry and his father sitting so happily together, it triggered my personal Demons of Unlovability, Isolation, and Helplessness in a big way. I felt my gut sink, I felt like I was suffocating and like I had to get out of there.

2. How could I have held space for that emotion?

When I felt that emotional flooding, it would have been more helpful to recognize that and just say something like, "Wow. I can feel something happening in me right now," and notice that reaction. In that circumstance, had I stopped and said that I was being flooded with emotion, I know that Jerry and his father would have been very understanding and want to support me. But, even if I didn't tell them what I was experiencing, but instead told them that I had to use the restroom, I could have taken a few moments in private to notice and hold space for my extreme emotional reaction.

3. What could I have asked my triggered demon?

Looking back on that experience, I know exactly what would have happened had I been able to ask my personal Demons why they were reacting so strongly. I would have been flooded with a deep pain and sadness that my father simply had no interest in being involved in my life and how profoundly that impacted me.

4. What could I have said to the wounded part of myself?

In that moment, the pain of rejection and feelings of worthlessness were debilitating. Those wounded parts of myself needed to have those feelings validated, to hear that I am loved, and to know that I am not alone. So, I could have said something like this to my personal Demons:

> I totally understand why you are up right now. Seeing the love that Jerry and his father share is a harsh reminder of what you do not have from your own father. I want you to know, despite that, you are lovable and a lot of people care about you. This is not a reflection of you. I am here with you and will help take care of you.

Had I been able to recognize that I had been triggered and to speak to the wounded parts of myself in a compassionate and supportive way, my experience that night would have been very different. It would have been a moment of feeling triggered and some processing of those emotions, rather than repeating the same pattern of isolating myself and rejecting healthy people in my life.

Let's talk through another example.

Rejecting Another Relationship

Danielle is one of those women who seems to have it all. She is gorgeous, brilliant, and articulate, and she has an interpersonal style that is disarming and sweet. Most guys would see her as an ideal partner, and she would love to be in a relationship. Yet, her struggle to form a stable intimate relationship has been a major source of frustration for her.

In one of our sessions, Danielle described a date she had the previous weekend with a man who she really liked. She said the date was wonderful and she had a great time with him. She was excited that the two of them seemed so compatible, and she was looking forward to seeing where their relationship would go. The morning after their date, he sent her a text message to invite her to do something with him a couple days later. When she received his message, something happened. She felt herself starting to panic and was overtaken by an urgency to run away. Instead of responding with "yes, I would love that," she withdrew and didn't respond. When she finally responded, her tone was very different, and she told him she wanted to stay home instead of going out with him. He was bewildered by what he sensed as a sudden shift in her interest in him. This was followed by an unhelpful series of text exchanges between the two of them that ended with him saying that he was no longer interested in pursuing a relationship with her.

Danielle was devastated and became flooded with feelings of shame and failure. It felt like one more example in a string of failed relationships that had one element in common: her. The floodgates of self-judgment opened up, and she was swamped by feelings of being broken and unlovable. She simmered in a toxic soup of self-hate for several days afterward.

So what happened? Danielle had a trauma response where one of her personal demons kicked her out of the driver's seat and took over steering her emotions and behavior. The moment before her date's text, she was excited about a relationship with him. The moment after his text, she became a powerless spectator as she felt herself pull away and watched helplessly as another opportunity for an intimate relationship disappeared.

Now, let's walk through her experience to see how she could have navigated this situation differently.

1. What was her inflection point?

In Danielle's case, something happened to her when she received the follow-up text from the guy she liked. The moment she read the text, she felt something shift and she began to panic.

2. How could she have held space for her reaction?

When she felt that shift from reading his text, she could have paused for a moment and brought her attention to what she was feeling. It may have been helpful for her to imagine creating some kind of space where she could hold that emotional trigger and just notice her reaction.

3. What could she have asked her triggered demon?

Given Danielle's history with panicking when people get too close to her, she could have asked her wounded self why it was so frightened right now. Why was it trying to get her attention? She could have then simply sat with that question to see what images or messages emerged.

4. What could she have said to the wounded part of herself?

Because there was no reason for her to panic just because someone she was dating and who she liked wanted to get together with her again, she could have said something like this to the wounded part of herself:

> I know you are afraid of being hurt right now because you have been hurt and abandoned in the past. You are going to be okay. You don't need to be frightened. I will protect you and make sure that you are safe.

Had Danielle been able to navigate through her emotional response differently, she may still be in that relationship today. Interestingly, she recognized in the moment that something had been triggered when she received his text, but she didn't know how to navigate through her reaction in a more controlled and intentional way. So, her old pattern of pulling away from people when they get emotionally close took over, and she ended up alone again.

Reparenting Your Demons

If you want to move your demons out of the driver's seat of your life and learn how to have a different relationship with your wounded parts, here are some questions to answer for yourself:

1. Which demons seem to have the greatest influence in my life?
2. When do they tend to show up?
3. When I experience an emotional inflection point, how will I use these four steps of:
   a. Recognizing when I experience an emotional inflection point and pausing for a moment to experience what I am feeling.
   b. Creating a space where I can hold that wounded part of myself.
   c. Asking why this particular demon has been triggered and what it is trying to tell me.
   d. Reparenting my demon by validating the distress, assuring it that it is okay, and telling it that I will protect it.

Being able to recognize when the wounded parts are becoming triggered and going through the four steps to comfort and reparent them is an important part of healing our core self-concept. By intervening when emotions first become triggered, we can avoid hours of being stuck in emotional distress and all that goes with it. By reparenting our wounded parts, we can give them the validation and support they need in order to heal.

We can also do this with our partner if we are in a committed relationship where we can communicate to our partner when a wounded part of ourselves is being triggered. Although we still have to hold space for that wounded part of ourselves, our partner can ask what the demon is trying to tell us and also give us the kind of validation and support that we didn't get in childhood. When couples learn how to do this for each other, it can be a very powerful way to build an emotional connection and develop great communication skills.

Every Day:
Your Daily Recovery Journal

Now let's turn our attention to a practice that we can do every day to help heal our core self-concept, regardless of whether we are triggered. I call this the Daily Recovery Journal, but if you would like to call it something else, that is totally fine.

As we did when processing emotional inflection points, we are going to pay attention to three things: negative feelings, distorted perceptions, and unhealthy behaviors. But instead of attending to those things in the present moment when we are experiencing them, we are going to reflect back on those experiences when they are no longer actively affecting us. By doing a daily journal, we will begin to recognize patterns in how our wounded parts show up in our lives, develop strategies for avoiding being triggered, and create a healthier narrative around our overall experience in life.

Getting Started

Starting your Daily Recovery Journal is pretty simple. All you need is a standard-size spiral-bound notebook, a pen, and a private place where you can write. Here is what to do:

1. Set aside a time to write your journal. It is probably best to do this at the end of the day. Plan to spend between ten to fifteen minutes. You will use one page per day.

2. At the top of the page, write the date, the two or three wounded parts of yourself that tend to get triggered, and then three words: Feelings, Perceptions, and Behaviors. For example, the top of your page may look something like this:

   June 9, 2025   Worthlessness, Isolation, Helplessness
   Feelings, Perceptions, and Behaviors

3. In the evening, review your day and reflect on whether any of these particular demons showed up in your life, and if so, how. It may be good to be very specific about what happened to trigger those feelings. For example, we may write something like, "When I couldn't get an issue figured out at work, I suddenly felt like a total failure and started to flood with negative feelings about myself."

4. Next, expand on the the feelings, perceptions, and behaviors that were triggered. For example, you may write something like, "It felt like I was the only one who was struggling. I thought to myself that everyone else could do their job just fine. Why can't I? I felt very exposed as if everyone could tell that I was a failure and actually considered quitting and finding another job."

5. Now let's pretend that there was an "Ideal You" that was in that situation. The "You" that did not struggle with wounded parts of themselves. What would that Ideal You say to the you that was struggling? This may be something like, "The fact that you struggled with the situation at work has nothing to do with you. The issue that you are struggling with is a problem for a lot of people. You are fully capable and respected at work. Although you may feel like a failure, it just isn't true."

6. Next, think about how you could have responded differently. What could you have said or done differently that

would have made the situation better? How could you have processed through your emotional response differently so that you had a clearer understanding of what was happening? Write all of that down. It is important not to beat yourself up about the way you did respond. This exercise is merely to look at some alternative ways of responding in the future.

7. Lastly, look for opportunities to apologize or correct situations where you may have said or did things that were unfair or hurtful to others. Did we lash out in frustration to our partner or coworkers? Did we disappear from work when others were relying on us? Did we engage in any self-destructive behaviors? There is no judgment on that. We just need to get it down on paper and look at it and then action when appropriate. We need to have the courage to take accountability for our behavior, even if it was clearly the result of being triggered. After all, accountability is the prerequisite to forgiveness.

If we do this inventory consistently, a very clear pattern of how our trauma responses show up will emerge. In most cases, we will see that it's one or two triggers that seem to get us in trouble. Most of us notice that by doing this daily exercise, we better recognize when we are becoming triggered, and since we have written down what we should do in those circumstances, over time will are more successful in navigating those situations.

Moving Forward

Healing your core self-concept is entirely possible, but it takes some time. The process is also very different from what you learned in the previous chapter about how to calm your emotions. Whereas the goal of calming your emotions centered around getting your brain out of the alarm response and processing trauma memories into long-term memory, the goal here is to recognize when wounds to our sense of self become triggered and heal them through a process of reparenting them.

Again, this all takes time and persistence. Healing from the effects of emotional trauma is not fast, particularly when you are dealing with wounded parts of your self-concept. Remember, healing is a process, not a destination. Focus on what is right in front of you each day and try to navigate each moment the best you can. If you continue showing up and applying the tools you are learning here, you will soon notice a significant difference in how you feel.

CHAPTER 9

Strengthening Your Relationships

CREATING AND MAINTAINING STABLE intimate relationships is often a challenge for those of us who have experienced emotional trauma. The reason is that the foundation of all healthy relationships is the ability for two partners to emotionally attune to each other and remain connected, even during times of conflict. Emotional trauma can make this difficult in a few ways. First, one of the effects of emotional trauma is the emotional dysregulation from unprocessed trauma experiences. Having our brain stuck in the alarm response and experiencing emotional outbursts, dissociation, numbing, flashbacks, and other trauma effects can make it very difficult to remain emotionally attuned to our partner. Second, our damaged sense of self will create relationship challenges as well, particularly during conflict, when our personal wounds become triggered and our feelings, thoughts, and actions become hijacked by our personal demons. Third, by growing up in a home where we did not have a healthy connection with our parents, and our parents often did not have healthy relationships themselves, we often enter into adulthood with unhealthy attachment styles that can get in the way of us forming healthy attachment bonds with our partner.

Because of these challenges, we have to be more intentional about how we navigate through our relationships than those who do not have a history of emotional trauma. We have to look for ways to remain emotionally connected and engaged with our partner, even when we are struggling ourselves. We also have to be more intentional in how we communicate so that we can avoid saying or doing things that may trigger a trauma response in either ourselves or our partner, and learn how to de-escalate situations that become emotionally heated. We have to understand how our own attachment challenges may affect how we connect with our partner and intentionally foster a healthier attachment style in our relationships. I know that this sounds like a lot, but if you apply the information and skills that you are learning in this book, there is no reason why you cannot be successful.

Communication Is the Key

The key idea in this chapter is that building strong relationships and repairing after conflict really comes down to how we communicate. Communication is the conduit through which relationships are formed and maintained, and is the primary mechanism by which we either draw closer to our partner or push them away. When we use the word *communication*, we are referring to all of the ways that we send messages to our partner, whether it is through the words that we say, how we respond to their bids for connection, the tone of our voice, how attentive we are, and whether we are emotionally present in the relationship. All of these verbal and nonverbal cues impact the emotional tone of the relationship and shape the way in which we attune to each other.

This chapter is about exploring ways in which communication affects our relationships, particularly intimate relationships with a committed partner. We will discuss how communication affects our five existential needs and the effect on our core self-concept, and how primary and secondary emotions affect the ways in which we communicate. We will then talk about the Rules of Communication Hygiene, which are important guidelines for effective emotional communication. Lastly, we will discuss the Emotional Check-In Exercise that I use with all of my clients as a framework for communicating differently.

Communication and Our Five Existential Needs

If we look at why certain messages tend to draw us together, while others tend to push us apart, we will find the difference lies in how they impact the five existential needs of our core self-concept. You recall from previous chapters that we all have five basic existential needs:

- The need for a sense of identity
- The need for a sense of connection
- The need for a sense of safety
- The need for a sense of value
- The need for a sense of agency

Just about every conflict that I see in my practice centers around one of these needs. Let's take a quick look at each of them.

The Need for a Sense of Identity: Do I Feel Like I Can Be My Authentic Self with You?

We need to feel like we are accepted for who we are, and not feel like we have to be some variant of ourselves that our partner will find acceptable. We need to feel like we are allowed to be our goofy and imperfect selves without feeling judged, shamed, or mocked. We need to feel that who we are as our authentic selves is loved and supported. If we don't feel that way, we will tend to shut parts of ourselves down and internalize self-shame. We will struggle with self-doubt and may feel like we need to check with our partner to make sure that what we want to do is acceptable to them. Over time, we can lose our sense of self to some degree and feel as though there is a part of us that remains hidden.

The Need for a Sense of Connection: Do I Feel Like You Are Here with Me?

We need to feel like our partner is here with us, particularly during times when we are upset. When we feel like our partner is present, we tend to feel a sense of stability and vibrance in the relationship and that we are moving through life as a partnership. If we feel like our partner is not emotionally present or is checked out of the relationship, it will tend to trigger feelings of panic, loneliness, and emptiness, or we may become hypercritical of them in an attempt to get them reengaged. We may feel like it is our responsibility to do everything on our own, feel unsupported, and even get to a point where we resign ourselves to the fact that we will live the rest of our lives feeling alone.

The Need for a Sense of Safety:
Do I Feel Like I Can Trust You with My Wellbeing?

We need to feel that our partner is a safe harbor for us where we can relax, be vulnerable, and feel protected. We need to have a sense of trust that our partner is going to be there for us and have our back when the times get tough, that we can take risks with them without fear of being hurt. We need to have a sense that emotional or physical violence toward us by our partner is so detached from reality that it would be unthinkable. Unfortunately, betrayals of trust, verbal or physical aggression, shaming, blaming, and inconsistency can all undermine our sense of safety with our partner. When this happens, we may struggle with trust and feel as though a part of us is always on guard.

The Need for a Sense of Value:
Do I Feel Like I Matter to You?

We all have a need to feel seen, validated, and that we matter to our partner. We need to feel like our partner notices us, values spending time with us, and desires to be close to us. In essence, we need to have a sense that we exist in the heart of our partner and that we are important to them. When our partner seems preoccupied, doesn't seem to pick up on our signals that we are distressed, or seems to ignore us, we can feel very unloved, like we don't matter, and can really struggle with feelings of worthlessness, being unappreciated, and that we are somehow "not enough" for them. If we don't feel valued by our partner, we may have a sense that it doesn't matter if we are even in the relationship and we may engage in affairs or other behaviors in order to feel valued or to punish our partner for not noticing us.

The Need for a Sense of Agency: Do I Feel Like You Help Me Accomplish My Dreams?

We all need to have a sense of being an active agent in our own relationship. We need to feel as though we are in a collaborative partnership and are not just a passive companion in our partner's life. There is a part of us who has dreams about what we would like to accomplish in life, and having a partner who will help support us in those dreams and be an active participant is very important. If we feel like we have no sense of agency in the relationship, that our ideas aren't good enough, or that no matter what we do, we cannot effect change, then there will tend to be a part of us that may become resentful, or we may simply give up trying and emotionally shut down.

Speaking Directly to the Five Needs

An important question to ask ourselves when we are trying to establish and maintain a healthy relationship is how the messages that we send to our partner speaks to their five needs.

- Are we communicating in a way that makes them feel accepted for who they are?
- Are we letting them know that we are emotionally present with them?
- Are we demonstrating that our partner can trust us with their vulnerability?
- Are we communicating that we see them and value them?
- Are we sending messages to our partner that we support their goals and dreams?

If you want to see how much speaking directly to these needs matters, try saying something like this to your partner and see how they respond:

I just want you to know that even though I may not always say it, I really appreciate who you are, you have a big presence in my heart, and I am so happy that you are a part of my life. I want you to know that your happiness matters a lot to me, I am here to support you, and I will always have your back when times get tough.

If you say it sincerely, your partner will be affected by hearing what you said. If they are not used to hearing things like this from you, they may nervously laugh or question whether you have lost your mind. That's okay. Just let your partner have that response. Deep down, your message will still be heard and will affect how they feel. If they have longed to hear something like this from you, they may cry or tell you how much that means to them.

Of course, we also need to hear these things from our partner as well. It is entirely okay to need to hear that you matter to them, that you are safe, that they are present with you, and that they accept and support who you are. There is nothing wrong with writing down the statement above, handing it to your partner, and saying, "This is what I need to hear from you."

Asking for what you need from your partner does not negate the legitimacy of their response. Many times our partners may hold us dear to their heart, but simply not have the language to express it in a way that would be helpful to us. As long as our partner could read the paragraph above and honestly say, "yes, I feel all of that for you," then it is okay for them to just read it to you so they can practice their own communication skills, and for you not to reject what they are saying simply because they had to say "I love you" from a cue card. We all have to start somewhere.

Conflict Centered around the Five Needs

If the way in which partners communicate with each other does not support these five needs, a pattern of conflict will tend to arise centered around the unmet need. A sign that this may be happening is when conflict seems to emotionally escalate for no apparent reason, and what should have been a simple conversation may suddenly feel impossible to resolve.

I would invite you (and your partner, if you currently have one) to reflect on some recent conflicts and see if you can identify which of these unmet needs was at the core of the arguments. If you don't currently have a partner, reflect on conflicts from your most recent past relationship to identify which needs drove the arguments. For example, if you and your partner had a heated argument about something like who to invite for a holiday dinner, what drove the emotional escalation of the conflict was probably not about who was going to be eating your turkey. There was something else driving the escalation. Most of the time, we will find that we were feeling unheard, dismissed, unsafe, powerless, or some other emotion related to one of our five existential needs not being met.

If you spend a little time to do this exercise and take a sober look at what emotional experiences tend to get triggered during conflict, you will likely find a pattern where the arguments that seem to escalate the most tend to center around one or two of these unmet needs. If you don't see the connection yet between your pattern of conflict and these five needs, that's okay. Just remain open to observing the emotions that tend to show up during conflict. Recognizing your pattern can be an important first step to creating an off-ramp when it feels like things are starting to escalate.

Next, let's discuss another important topic that will help us navigate relationships more effectively. That is understanding how communicating from a primary emotion or a secondary emotion affects our emotional connection with our partner.

Primary Emotions and Secondary Emotions

Emotions like anger, panic, or becoming overwhelmed and shutting down don't just happen on their own. We experience these because something triggered them. In other words, there was some earlier event that preceded a secondary rush of distress. The original emotional trigger, called a primary emotion, happened when we perceived or experienced something that felt threatening or hurtful in some way. When we felt threatened or hurt, the emotional circuits in our brain created a response that was intended to help us cope with the perceived threat. This secondary response is often in the form of the fight, flight, freeze, or fawn response, but may also involve reactions from wounded parts of our self-concept, such as feelings of worthlessness, helplessness, self-shame, or dissociation.

For example, if someone cuts us off in traffic, we usually have an initial sinking feeling of fear when we first notice them pulling in front of us. This is the primary response. Very quickly afterward, we will have a secondary emotion. In this type of circumstance, it will likely be part of the alarm response. So, we may either become angry, panic and freeze, or try to avoid them.

Whether we are in traffic or having a conversation with our partners, this secondary response can happen so quickly following the primary emotion that we may not even notice the primary emotion at all. We may just notice the sudden flood of rage that seemed to come out of nowhere. But, if we could slow everything down and look at what is happening inside our emotional system, we will notice that an emotional inflection point occurred at one point that was quickly followed by a secondary emotional response. That emotional inflection point is the moment that the primary emotion was triggered and we felt threatened, unsafe, unheard, dismissed, abandoned, or some other impingement on a wounded part of ourselves. The secondary emotion is everything that came after that, and it is the brain's attempt to cope with a perceived threat to our well-being by either distancing ourselves or going on the offensive.

Understanding this distinction between the primary emotion and secondary emotion is very important because it determines how interpersonal conflict will tend to unfold. The human mind is wired to respond empathetically when someone is afraid or hurt. We naturally want to engage them and comfort them. You see this all the time when strangers stop to help someone who is wounded, help a lost child, or comfort someone who is upset. So, when we can communicate to our partner that we are feeling hurt, sad, empty, or alone, it will tend to elicit a compassionate response from them and draw them closer to us.

The human mind is also wired to respond with defensiveness when someone is aggressive, shaming, or threatening. There is a natural fight-or-flight response that is triggered when someone is displaying obnoxious, accusatory, demeaning, or rageful behavior. Therefore, when we communicate to our partner from an angry or shaming place, we will tend to elicit a defensive response from them and push them further away from us.

When we can stay in our primary emotion and communicate our hurt or fear with our partner during a period of conflict, we will have a good chance of finding resolution and repair without the argument escalating out of control. However, when we get stuck in our secondary emotion and communicate our anger or blame, the argument will tend to escalate out of control, and it will be much harder to find any resolution.

So, the key points here to remember are:

- When we can communicate from the place of our primary emotion, we will tend to elicit an empathetic response from our partner, and they will tend to become more emotionally engaged with us.

- When we communicate from the place of our secondary emotion, we will tend to elicit a defensive response from our partner, and they will tend to become less emotionally engaged with us.

Write this down. Tape it to your refrigerator door. Say it to yourself a hundred times in the mirror. Tattoo it on your forehead. Do whatever you need to do to remember this because it is the key to navigating through emotional conversations effectively.

Next, let's take what we learned about the five core-self concept needs, primary and secondary emotion, and how these show up in relationships to create some rules for effective communication. I call these the Rules of Communication Hygiene.

The Rules of Communication Hygiene

Most people have experienced times when attempts to resolve a disagreement only seem to make the problem worse. During these times, it seems that no matter what is said, how much the partners try to explain themselves to each other or ask the other partner why they are so upset, it just feels like adding gasoline to the flames. Partners may feel overwhelmed, frustrated, agitated, and stuck. If this continues long enough, partners may say things to each other that may feel real in the moment but that they later regret, and eventually simply shut down and go their separate ways. Instead of finding resolution, the partners are often left feeling helpless, exhausted, alone, and sad.

Couples who love and care about each other can suddenly find themselves embroiled in a conflict that escalates out of control despite their best efforts. It is tragic to watch because in their attempt to bond with each other and resolve an issue, they employ a series of communication strategies that do just the opposite; they push the other person away. We just discussed how communicating from a place of secondary emotion tends to cause an escalation in conflict and pushes partners away from each other, but there are other ways that we communicate that can have the same effect. If a pattern of disconnection happens enough, each partner will begin to develop a layer of "emotional scar tissue" that makes full reconciliation even more difficult to achieve.

Several years ago, I developed a set of communication guidelines to help my clients navigate through emotional conversations more effectively. This set of guidelines helps couples navigate emotional or difficult conversations without escalation and allows each partner to remain engaged. The basic premise is that when couples feel as though their partner is emotionally engaged and fully present with them during difficult conversations, each partner tends to feel heard and held in a safe space. When this happens, couples can negotiate meaningful and satisfying solutions to their disagreements. The intent of thes rules is to find ways of interacting during times of distress that allow both partners to remain actively engaged with each other.

Rule 1. It Is Always Safe to Communicate State

This communication technique is all about sharing with your partner what you are experiencing in the moment. In other words, if you were to stick an emotional thermometer into your gut right now, what would it read? Stressed? Sad? Angry? Hurt? Lonely? Frustrated?

Communicating your emotional state in a completely nonjudgmental and nonaccusatory way communicates to them that you are emotionally present and engaged. It is communicating a primary emotion that will tend to elicit an empathetic response from your partner, rather than an adversarial one. Being able to communicate state is one of the easiest and most important tools you can use during any difficult conversation.

For example, if your partner is telling you what a rough day they had at work, you may feel a sense of tension in your own gut as an empathetic response to hearing their experience. If we were to respond by communicating our current state, we could say something like, "Wow. I can feel myself getting tense just hearing about what you are going through."

If your partner tells you how frustrated they are that you forgot to do something that you said you were going to do, you may have a primary emotion of embarrassment, regret, or even self-shame. If you were to do a quick gut check and communicate state, you may respond with something like, "I feel very bad about disappointing you" or "I am very sorry. I feel embarrassed right now."

None of these statements is passing any judgment on either ourselves or our partner. It is simply an exercise in taking a measurement in the emotional tone in our gut and speaking it out loud.

Rule 2. Explore, Rather than Explain

When you explore, you are engaging your partner in an effort to better understand what they are experiencing. If your partner says, "I am very upset," you can engage them by asking questions such as, "What is going on?" or "What are you experiencing right now?" The intent is simply to understand what your partner is experiencing from a place of compassionate curiosity. When asked questions like these, your partner will likely feel that you are interested in their experience, that you value them, and that you are fully present in the moment.

When you explain, you are disconnecting from your partner's experience and trying to defend yourself or avoid having to deal with your own emotional discomfort. This usually happens when we feel blamed or responsible for our partner's distress. So, instead of engaging with them and being present with their experience, we try to explain ourselves, challenge whether what they are feeling is legitimate, or try to fix them so they are no longer upset. Unfortunately, this is not helpful because when we explain, we are making it all about us and not about our partner's distress.

Explaining, rather than exploring, is one of the primary forces that keeps couples stuck in an escalating spiral about who is more right about a situation, who remembers things the correct way, or who is more at fault in a situation, when the real thing that they both seek is to feel heard, appreciated, and connected. Explaining is driven by an urgency to get our partner to understand us, rather than us focusing on understanding our partner. Unfortunately, the result is that neither partner ends up feeling understood.

The key to this rule of emotional hygiene is to put your attention into the heart of your partner in an effort to understand what they are experiencing without judgment, and simply allowing them to have their experience rather than getting them to understand your point.

Rule 3. Never Speak for Your Partner's Emotions

When your partner is upset, there is a tendency to name the emotion for them. For example, if your partner looks upset, you might say something like, "Wow, aren't you in a bad mood?" or during a disagreement ask, "Why are you so angry?" Most of us have made comments like this and have seen what happens. Does it make the other person feel better or worse? Almost invariably, when you make a statement about what your partner is feeling, it escalates the situation.

The rule here is to observe and explore. Asking, "Are you in a bad mood right now?" feels very different from "Why are you in such a bad mood?" Saying, "You look very upset right now, are you angry?" feels very different from asking, "Why are you angry?" The difference is subtle, but important. In the first instance we're calling on our partner to share with us what they are experiencing, which feels interested and engaged. When we name our partner's emotion, even if we are correct, we are not emotionally engaging. When you observe that your partner appears upset and want to understand what they are feeling, you are engaging them.

When you name the emotion for them, your partner doesn't feel engaged. They tend to feel judged.

Rule 4. Don't Try to Manage the Emotions of the Other Person

Trying to manage the emotional life of another person can take two different forms. One is to "mother them" by trying to make them feel better. The other is to not say things that may upset them. When you do either of these, you are essentially taking over and trying to do the emotional work for the other person. An example of this is a family that needs to be very careful not to say the wrong thing around an alcoholic father so he doesn't fly off into a rage. Another example would be feeling like you have to take responsibility to make sure that your mentally ill mother doesn't become too upset and emotionally collapse. In less extreme examples, you may decide not to communicate about your own struggles and need for support from your partner because they may become defensive and shut down, or you may feel like you always have to attend to your partner's needs to the detriment of your own.

In any of these cases, trying to manage the emotional life of another person by suppressing your own needs or distress does quite a bit of damage to a relationship over time. There is commonly a loss of a sense that your partner is a safe, nurturing, and supportive person for you, as well as a loss of trust. Sharing your emotional experience and needs with your partner is a critical element of a healthy emotional bond. Both partners need to take accountability for their own reactions.

Most people can tell when they are starting to manage the emotions of the other person. There is usually a sense of urgency to jump in and rescue their feelings. When we feel that happening, the best thing to do is to stop, notice what we are experiencing, and ask ourselves why we feel the need to be the hero here.

Why can't we just let them have their experience without our needing to manage them? While you don't need to be insensitive, it is important that you speak your truth and let the other person do the best they can to manage their own emotions.

Rule 5. Take Accountability for Your Side of the Street

Accountability is the prerequisite to forgiveness. When we do something dumb or act like an ass, the first step to healing our relationship with others is being able to fully take accountability for our actions and how they affected our partner. People have a surprising capacity to forgive and move forward, but that can only happen when we acknowledge our behavior and how it affected the other person, and what action we will take in the future to avoid a similar situation.

People respect those who can take accountability because it demonstrates maturity, courage, and the presence of a moral compass. This is particularly important when it comes to relationships, because maintaining a healthy emotional bond requires a shared sense of what is real. If someone is unable to be accountable, it forces others to pretend that hurtful words or actions didn't happen. Relationships then become based on a make-believe reality where authentic connection and communication is replaced by partners having to suppress their own needs and withdrawing from engagement. Taking accountability doesn't have to be an exercise in self-flagellation, it just needs to be an acknowledgment of what we did and a desire to repair our relationship. It can be something as simple as "I apologize for saying what I did. It was unfair, and I'm sorry for that. What would be helpful right now?"

Rule 6. Agree On an Emotional Fire Escape Plan

During my initial sessions with clients, I have them choose a phrase that they can say to each other when emotions are starting to escalate and they want to put a pause on a conversation until things cool down a bit. These agreements have three parts:

1. Communicating your own personal emotional state, not your partner's, with your chosen phrase. Remember, we can't speak for our partner's emotional experience.

2. Asking for a temporary pause in the conversation, and both parties agreeing to honor that request.

3. Committing to resume the conversation within a reasonable time period—20 minutes, an hour, or later in the day. It is best not to let the conversation go unresolved overnight if possible.

Typically, these are phrases like, "I am starting to feel myself escalating, and I need to take a break. Can we talk about this after dinner?" or, "I am losing my objectivity, and I would like to ask that we take a pause. Can we come back to this conversation in a little while?" Even something like, "I am freaking out a bit right now and need to stop. Can we talk later?" is okay as long as both partners have agreed on the language.

The time to create your fire escape plan is not when your house is on fire. It needs to be done in a collaborative way during a period of calm so that everyone knows what to do when an emergency arises and panic sets in. It's the same way here. You need an emotional fire escape plan before emotions start escalating. Having a phrase that each partner can agree to honor as a way to pause the situation can be extremely helpful in avoiding unnecessary distress and harm.

A Simple Communication Pattern

Let's take a look at what a pattern of communication might look like if we were to focus our communication on primary emotion, include language that supports our five existential needs, and follow the rules of communication hygiene. This is an easy pattern that I teach my clients and have them practice every day. Here is a short exercise that you can do with a partner. It only has a few steps and is not that difficult. It just takes practice. Here are the steps:

1. Communicate state
2. Seek understanding
3. Explore the experience
4. Offer support

Find a time each day where the two of you can spend five minutes to do this exercise. It is best to do it when you won't be disturbed by kids, pets, the TV, or the phone. Also, don't do it right before bed. Let's take a look at each of these steps individually.

If you are not currently in a partnership, take note of these concepts. It will still be helpful to understand the principles of communication hygiene so that you can use these techniques when you are in a committed relationship.

Step 1. Communicate State

The goal of this step is to sit down across from each other and simply verbalize what emotion you are feeling in the moment. That's it. Just one or two words.

What words should you say?

Remember that emotional thermometer in your gut? What does it say? These could be things like "frustrated," "happy," "hopeful," "angry," "tense," or whatever feels accurate. Words like "tired," "okay," and "fine," are not emotions, so those don't count. If you have trouble labeling the emotion that you are feeling, pay attention to body sensations in your gut and chest and describe those. "Tightness in my gut" and "heaviness in my chest" are sensations associated with emotion, whereas words like "I'm alright" are not.

So, just sit down across from your partner, look at your emotional thermometer, and read what it says about your emotional state. Next, tell your partner what you are feeling in the moment in a matter-of-fact way. That's it. Don't explain why you feel that way, or elaborate at all. Just one sentence, like this:

"I feel nervous right now."
"I am feeling hopeful."
"I am really angry."

The key to this part of the exercise is the process of mentally checking in with your gut and saying out loud what is happening emotionally in the moment. What you felt like earlier doesn't matter. What you have felt like in general doesn't matter. All that matters is what you are experiencing as you sit there doing this exercise. Don't elaborate on what you are feeling or justify what you are feeling. This first step is just about communicating state.

Step 2. Seek Understanding

Once you communicate your emotional state, it is your partner's turn to respond. For this exercise, the only responses allowed are ones that elicit more information from you. This can be in the form of questions or statements such as:

"Can you say more?"
"Tell me more about what is going on."
"Help me understand what you are experiencing."

The key is for your partner to invite you to share more as a way of engaging with your experience so they can understand what is emotionally going on in the moment. In this step, your partner should never ask "why" questions, even though it is very tempting. "Why" questions get you out of a collaborative space and into a place where you are qualifying, defending, or justifying your experience. This step is all about exploring rather than explaining.

It is common for a partner to react to you stating that you feel angry, hurt, fearful, or sad, and to want some reassurance that your feelings are not about them. But they will just have to sit with that discomfort during the exercise. The point is to learn a new pattern of interaction where the two of you can stay in a collaborative space. If your partner hears what you say, and all of a sudden you have to reassure them, then you have shifted into a different dynamic.

Step 3. Explore the Experience

When your partner asks you to say more, this is your call to sit with the feelings in your gut and say more about what you are experiencing. It may be tempting for you to say something like:

"There really isn't anything else to say."

"I don't know what else to say about it."

But here is where digging in can really pay dividends for you. Reflect back on your gut again and try to come up with something else to say about the emotion you're feeling. It almost doesn't matter what it is. Does your anger have a color associated with it? Does your fear have a body sensation? Does the tightness in your chest have a sense of dread associated with it? Just sit with your feelings for a moment and see if you can come up with something else to share.

If you legitimately try, and you can't come up with something else to say, that's okay. The important part of this step is the process of sitting with your experience and trying to describe it in more detail. If there's nothing else there, just say something like:

"Nothing else is coming up."

Don't say anything about what triggered the feeling or what you plan to do about it. This exercise is simply about emotional communication, not problem-solving. There will be time to do all of the logical processing later. Right now, it's all about sitting with the emotional part.

Step 4. Offer Support

Once you do your best to share more about your experience, your partner asks if there is a way that they can offer some support to you. This can be something as simple as asking questions like:

"How can I be helpful right now?"
"What would be helpful from me?"

The goal for your partner is to communicate that they are there to support you. Again, this is about them being present, not offering their opinion. This can sometimes be hard because when you are upset, your partner may want to help fix things or withdraw.

A good rule when your partner asks how they can be helpful is to restrict your answer to how they can be helpful in this particular moment, not how they can be helpful in general. A bad answer here would be to launch into how your partner needs to be different in general in order to be supportive. For example, I have had clients do this exercise in session and when the partner who is trying to be supportive asks, "What would be helpful from me?", the other partner launches into a laundry list of all the things they are doing wrong in the relationship. If you do that, this whole exercise will derail. Just stick with what, if anything, would be helpful in the moment.

One you are done with this exercise, thank each other and go about your day.

A Simple Pattern with an Inflection Point

We introduced emotional inflection points in the previous chapter to describe the moment when there is a shift in our emotional tone from one state to another. Inflection points are valuable to recognize not only when trying to identify when a trauma reaction is happening within us, but also when trying to navigate through conflict without it escalating.

All of us have experienced a situation where a conversation starts out well, but ends up in a fight. When this happens, people often feel a sense of bewilderment about how things ended up going so badly so quickly. If we had a video recording of the conversation from start to finish, and could slow it down, we would see a point in the conversation where one partner or the other said something that caused a shift in the tone of the conversation. Once that shift in tone occured and emotions begin to escalate, the fight-or-flight response and trauma reactions join the dance and make resolution very difficult.

A very important skill in communication is to recognize the moment that an inflection point happens and to pause the conversation to explore what happened. You could say something like this:

1. You (communicating state): "What just happened there? I felt the tone shift in the conversation. Did you notice that?"

2. Partner (communicating state): "Yeah, I did. I guess I started feeling really angry."

3. You (explore, rather than explain): "Was there something that I said to trigger that?"

4. Partner (communicating primary emotion): "Not something you said, but it felt like you weren't hearing what I was saying."

5. You (take accountability): "Okay. I apologize for that. I do want to hear what you are saying. Can we start from there?"

6. Partner: "Sure."

7. You (explore, rather than explain): "Help me understand what you were trying to say."

Although this was a simple example, the point is that using the rules of communication hygiene will help us navigate through conversations more effectively, even when a secondary emotion gets triggered and shifts the emotional tone of the conversation. All we have to do is bring it back to the inflection point and ask about the primary emotion that was triggered. Simply taking an objective look at what happened during the inflection point without judging who is right or wrong is a very important skill. What gets in the way for most people when they try this is that they feel such a need to be right that they simply cannot even hear what their partner is saying.

It is important to avoid saying things like, "I get what you are saying, but…," and then launching into your side of the argument. If you do, you are violating Rule 2, Explore, Rather than Explain, and the conversation will escalate. A better response after listening to your partner is to say something like, "So, where do we go from here?," to engage them in problem-solving.

When exploring inflection points, forget about who is right and who is wrong. That is not what you are trying to accomplish. The goal is to create clarity about what happened and for both you and your partner to work collaboratively to find a solution, even if that means taking a break and reconnecting later once emotions settle down.

Moving Forward

Working on our communication skills so that we can improve emotional connection in our relationships is different from the work we did in the previous couple of chapters. The work we did in the Calming Your Emotions chapter focused on becoming more grounded in our body and processing our trauma memories so we could shift our limbic system out of a constant state of alarm. The work we did in the Healing Your Core Self-Concept chapter focused on recognizing when wounds to our sense of self become triggered and how to heal the wounded parts of our self-concept. In this chapter our work is primarily on developing some new communication skills to help us form and maintain intimate connections with those who we love. Although the discussion in this chapter focused on communicating with intimate partners, we can apply these skills to other relationships as well, such as with family or friends.

We covered a lot in this chapter. Don't expect to be able to implement all of this immediately. Recovering from emotional trauma simply takes some time and persistence. It is entirely okay to focus on some parts of our discussion for a time and focus on other parts later. For example, you may want to work on implementing speaking directly to people's five existential needs. Once you have that down, you could focus on identifying your primary emotional responses and communicating those. Remember that recovery is a process and not a destination. If you focus on doing something small each day, your recovery journey will just become a normal part of your life.

CHAPTER 10

Your Journey of Recovery

CONGRATULATIONS ON MAKING IT to the last chapter! We have covered a lot of territory so far. We have introduced the concept of emotional trauma and talked about how it leads to emotional dysregulation, a damaged self-concept, and difficulty with relationships. We talked about the importance of having a holistic healing mindset for your journey of recovery, and we discussed specific ways to calm your emotions, heal your self-concept, and strengthen your relationships. Now it's time to take all that information and distill it into a plan of action that is right for you.

Everyone has their own life experience, unique personality, and different support system. Each of these shapes our personal experience with trauma and how it tends to show up in our mental, emotional, physical, sexual, and spiritual lives. Our goal now is to gain some clarity about where trauma is showing up in our lives, prioritize where to focus our energy and attention, and create a realistic and sustainable plan for our journey of recovery.

In step one, we will do a short self-evaluation to look at each area of our lives, and reflect on how much it is affected by emotional dysregulation, a damaged self-concept, and relationship difficulties. We can then use this information to craft our personal plan of action.

Self-Evaluation: How Is Emotional Trauma Affecting You?

In this simple self-evaluation, we will explore five areas of our lives—mental, emotional, physical, sexual, and spiritual—and rate how much we feel that emotional trauma is affecting that area. Using a scale of 0 to 10, with 0 being no impact and 10 being greatly impacted, please indicate the level of impact that you experience in each area of your life. For example, if the description captures your experience well, mark it a 10. If it does not resonate with your experience, mark it a 0. If it lies somewhere in between, then mark the level that best represents how much the statement reflects your experience.

Our Mental Life

Our mental life is the human experience of thought, understanding, strategizing, and contemplation. It is what allows us to make decisions, communicate ideas, interpret information from the world around us, and see ourselves objectively. Please rate how much you feel that emotional trauma is present in your mental life in these three ways:

- **Emotional Dysregulation:** Emotional dysregulation in our mental life tends to be experienced as difficulty in maintaining focus, feeling disorganized, scattered, and forgetful. We may struggle to manage our time effectively, experience racing thoughts, and may have been diagnosed with attention deficit disorder.

Presence in My Life: None   0 . . . . . 5 10   Significant

- **Damaged Self-Concept:** Damage to our self-concept in our mental life will typically affect how we perceive ourselves. We will tend to see ourselves as broken, flawed, helpless, or unlovable, and we will tend to interpret the events in our lives through that lens. We may feel like we have to guess at what normal is, and feel like things that are hard for us seem easy for others.

Presence in My Life: None   0 . . . . 5 10   Significant

- **Difficulty with Relationships:** Relationship difficulties in our mental life will tend to emerge from not having a good mental map of what a relationship should look like, a failure to recognize warning signs in unhealthy partners, and a lack of effective communication skills. We may hold unhealthy or unrealistic beliefs about relationships, and be rigid in our thinking.

Presence in My Life: None   0 . . . . 5 10   Significant

Our Emotional Life

Our emotional life is the human experience of feeling, attraction, joy, fear, love and other affective states. It is what organizes all of the input from our senses into a felt sense of having an experience, and it creates the feeling of being alive. Please rate how much you feel that emotional trauma is present in your emotional life in these three ways:

- **Emotional Dysregulation:** Emotional dysregulation in our emotional life tends to be experienced as sudden and intense swings in mood, irritability, emotional numbness, and experiencing heightened levels of anxiety, panic, or fear. We may experience flashbacks, nightmares, dissociation, or derealization.

Presence in My Life: None   0 . . . . 5 10   Significant

- **Damaged Self-Concept:** Damage to our self-concept in our emotional life will typically be experienced as being hypercritical of ourselves, feeling internalized shame, guilt, depression, or despair, and possibly feeling lost and rudderless. We may struggle to find ourselves, act impulsively, engage in people-pleasing behavior, feel like we don't belong, and struggle with addiction.

Presence in My Life: None   0 . . . . 5 10   Significant

- **Difficulty with Relationships:** Difficulty with relationships in our emotional life tends to manifest as a rapid increase in conflict intensity or the inability to calm down during an argument. We may become either hypercritical toward our partner, or emotionally shut down. We may experience feeling unheard, unseen, or unappreciated, and struggle to set boundaries.

Presence in My Life: None   0 . . . . 5 10   Significant

Our Physical Life

Our physical life is the human experience of physical presence. Our body is more than just a passive container for our soul. It is the source of all sensation and is deeply connected to the emotional circuits in the limbic system and brainstem. Please rate how much you feel that emotional trauma is present in your physical life in these three ways:

- **Emotional Dysregulation:** Emotional dysregulation in our physical life tends to show up in the body as physical manifestations of chronic stress, such as disrupted sleep patterns, high blood pressure, gastrointestinal distress, headaches, heart disease, sweating, rapid heart beat, panic attacks, or having a difficult time relaxing.

Presence in My Life: None   0 . . . . 5 10   Significant

- **Damaged Self-Concept:** Damage to our self-concept in our physical life will tend to affect how we hold ourselves (slumped vs. standing up straight), our comfort in making eye contact, personal hygiene, and health choices. It is common for people with emotional trauma to use food as an emotional management strategy, have body image issues, or struggle with anorexia.

Presence in My Life: None   0 . . . . 5 10   Significant

- **Difficulty with Relationships:** Difficulty with relationships in our physical life can show up as an aversion to physical touch, becoming tense during times of intimacy, feeling parts of our body go numb, sexual dysfunction, or painful intercourse. Physical intimacy may be experienced as distressing rather than enjoyable.

Presence in My Life: None   0 . . . . 5 10   Significant

Our Sexual Life

Our sexual life is the human experience of seeking pleasure, connection, desire, and affection, through the integration of imagination, physical touch, vulnerability, personal expression, and emotional bonding. Please rate how much you feel that emotional trauma is present in your sexual life in these three ways:

- **Emotional Dysregulation:** Emotional dysregulation in our sexual life may lead to an extreme in sexual interest, sudden emotional shifts during sex, high-risk sexual behavior, and a loss of self-control. Some may experience an intense and persistent sexual appetite, while others may feel a complete loss of sexual interest, even when they want to experience sexual desire.

    Presence in My Life: None   0 . . . . 5 10   Significant

- **Damaged Self-Concept:** Damage to our self-concept in our sexual life may manifest as significant emotional drops after sex where we feel a sense of sadness, anxiety, or emptiness, or using sex to feel a sense of closeness and value. Some may be drawn to nontraditional sex practices, such as kink or BDSM, as a form of self-therapy where they can reexperience traumatic events within a consensual context.

    Presence in My Life: None   0 . . . . 5 10   Significant

- **Difficulty with Relationships:** Difficulty with relationships in our sexual life can show up as conflict around a lack of sexual intimacy or a loss of a sense of closeness. On the other extreme, when one partner is in a hypersexual state, managing the extreme disparity in sexual appetite can be a real issue, particularly when there have been violations of trust.

    Presence in My Life: None   0 . . . . 5 10   Significant

Our Spiritual Life

Our spiritual life is the human experience of seeking meaning, higher purpose, and a sense of connection to something greater than ourselves, whether that be through a relationship with nature, religious faith, or a social movement. Please rate how much you feel that emotional trauma is present in your spiritual life in these three ways:

- **Emotional Dysregulation:** Emotional dysregulation in our spiritual life may show up as fanaticism about a particular spiritual movement, feeling that life is meaningless, or cycling through episodes of feeling connected to some higher purpose and then emotionally collapsing in a state of hopelessness and emptiness.

Presence in My Life: None   0 . . . . 5 10   Significant

- **Damaged Self-Concept:** Damage to our self-concept in our spiritual life will often manifest as a sense of meaninglessness and emptiness. There is often a sense that the world lacks any good, life is pointless, and nothing that we do ultimately matters. We may feel disconnected from our inner selves and may feel a constant sense of dread.

Presence in My Life: None   0 . . . . 5 10   Significant

- **Difficulty with Relationships:** Difficulty with relationships in our spiritual life will often be experienced as emotional disconnection from our partner arising from our own sense of emptiness. We may feel as though we don't have shared values with our partner, and we may find it hard to be emotionally present in the relationship.

Presence in My Life: None   0 . . . . 5 10   Significant

Our Life in General

Now that we have gone through each of the five different areas of our lives, let's do the same thing with our life in general. Please rate how much you feel that emotional trauma is generally present in your life in these three ways:

- **Emotional Dysregulation:** Emotional dysregulation is one of the hallmarks of acute trauma and is commonly experienced as being easily triggered, having difficulty soothing our emotions, feeling in a constant state of high alert, experiencing flashbacks, engaging in behaviors to avoid triggering situations, and experiencing the physical effects of chronic stress.

Presence in My Life: None   0 . . . . 5 10   Significant

- **Damaged Self-Concept:** Damage to our self-concept is commonly experienced as an internalized sense of shame, worthlessness, emptiness, unlovability, and feeling dirty and broken. We may struggle to find joy and suffer from chronic anxiety, depression, and hopelessness.

Presence in My Life: None   0 . . . . 5 10   Significant

- **Difficulty with Relationships:** Difficulty with relationships is commonly experienced by unstable emotional connections with a partner, conflict that tends to rapidly escalate, inability to repair after conflict, and a lack of a sense of intimacy. We may find ourselves emotionally shutting down or becoming hypercritical of our partner.

Presence in My Life: None   0 . . . . 5 10   Significant

Now that we have marked up each of these, let's move onto the next step in creating our plan, where we look at our scores and decide where to focus our healing work.

Prioritizing Your Focus

In this step, let's take the eighteen self-ranking scores from step one and look at them in a couple of ways. First, we will look at how emotional trauma may be affecting our emotions, self-concept, and relationships differently. Second, we will look at how emotional trauma may be affecting five areas of our life differently.

The Impact on Our Emotions, Self-Concept, and Relationships

Let's look at which of the three effects from emotional trauma seem to be the most present in our life. Add up each score from the Emotional Dysregulation, Damaged Self-Concept, and Difficulty with Relationships categories and place them on the scales below.

Emotional Dysregulation

    Score: _____   0 … 10 … 20 … 30 … 40 … 50 … 60

Damaged Self-Concept

    Score: _____   0 … 10 … 20 … 30 … 40 … 50 … 60

Difficulty with Relationships

    Score: _____   0 … 10 … 20 … 30 … 40 … 50 … 60

Now that you have added up your score and placed it on the scale:

- What do you notice?
- Is one of these areas much higher or lower than the others?
- What does this tell you about how emotional trauma may be impacting you in different ways?

The Impact in Different Areas of Our Life

Let's take a look at how emotional trauma may be showing up in different areas of your life. Add up the three numbers you have for each aspect of your life and place them on the scales below.

My Mental Life

    Score: _____　　　0 … 5 … 10 … 15 … 20 … 25 … 30

My Emotional Life

    Score: _____　　　0 … 5 … 10 … 15 … 20 … 25 … 30

My Physical Life

    Score: _____　　　0 … 5 … 10 … 15 … 20 … 25 … 30

My Sexual Life

    Score: _____　　　0 … 5 … 10 … 15 … 20 … 25 … 30

My Spiritual Life

    Score: _____　　　0 … 5 … 10 … 15 … 20 … 25 … 30

Now that you have added up your scores and placed them on the scale:

- What do you notice?
- Is one of these areas much higher or lower than the others?
- What does this tell you about how emotional trauma may be impacting the different areas of your life?

Reflecting on Your Experience

This self-evaluation exercise is not intended to diagnose you with anything. It is simply a tool to help you organize and clarify where you may be affected by emotional trauma. I encourage you to reflect on what this exercise showed you in conjunction with your day-to-day experience and write down one or two areas of your life that seem to be the greatest struggle for you. If you choose to do so, you may want to write those in your Daily Recovery Journal.

Creating a Plan

Now that we have reflected on the way in which emotional trauma can show up in our lives and have written down a couple of areas that are particularly difficult for us, we can turn our attention to creating a plan of action for moving forward. There are two parts to this. The first is to choose one or two areas that you want to prioritize during this part of your journey. Although you may be tempted to try to fix everything right now, that is unrealistic and may set you up for disappointment. For those of us who have been living with the effects of emotional trauma for many years, there is often a sense of urgency to heal ourselves as quickly as possible. But I encourage you to resist that temptation. The slow and methodical approach is the quickest path to healing.

The second part of this exercise is to create a vision of what a healthier version of yourself would look like. After all, if you do not have a picture in your head of how you would like your life to be better, how do you know if you are healing? Visualizing the perfect version of yourself also creates a guide that allows us to start intentionally acting as though we have already achieved healing.

Prioritizing Your Focus

When you are selecting the part or parts that you want to prioritize first, consider a couple of suggestions:

- If you are going to work on only one part of yourself that has been impacted the most by emotional trauma, then choose one of the big three: dysregulated emotions, damaged self-concept, or difficulty with relationships. These are the primary systems that are impacted by trauma. As we calm our emotions, heal our self-concept, and strengthen our relationships, everything else tends to improve along with them. It's like that old saying that a rising tide lifts all boats.

- If you are going to work on two areas, work on one of the big three, and then select one of areas of your life that you want to focus on as well: mental, emotional, physical, sexual, or spiritual. Although it is totally your choice what you work on, attending to either your physical health, spirituality, sexuality, or mental health while also working on calming your emotions, healing your self-concept, or strengthening your relationships tends to feel very good for a lot of people.

In general, it may be helpful to work on the big three in this order: dysregulated emotions, damaged self-concept, and then strengthening relationships—in the same order that we discussed them. Here is why. It will be very difficult to heal your self-concept if your brain is still stuck in a state of alarm and your emotions are dysregulated. However, once your emotions are stabilized a bit, you can make great progress on healing your self-concept. Similarly, being successful in building healthier relationships will be much more difficult if you are struggling with emotional dysregulation or being triggered by wounded parts of yourself. The three previous chapters describe many tools that you can use to heal these critical parts of yourself.

Providing specific tools to help you improve the five areas of your life is beyond what I can provide here. The reason is that these things are so highly personal that it would be impossible to guide you on what is right for your physical health, or what is right for your sex life, in the same way that I can guide you on how to heal the deeper circuits in the brain that are impacted by emotional trauma. What I do suggest is that you write down in your notebook what these areas would look like in the perfect version of yourself, and begin working toward that vision.

Visualize the Perfect Version of Yourself

Having a vision in mind of what a perfect version of you will look like is very helpful in giving you a guidepost to check your progress. Because we are dealing with your journey of recovery from emotional trauma, this perfect version of yourself should have three parts:

1. An emotional part
2. A self-concept part
3. A relationship part

Here are a few questions to consider when crafting a vision of what a more perfect you would look like. I suggest writing these down in your notebook and periodically looking back at them to check how you are doing. How does the perfect version of yourself:

- Set and hold boundaries?
- Handle conflict in relationships?
- Engage their sexuality?
- Feel about their value and lovability?
- Advocate for themselves?
- Deal with intense emotion when it arises?
- Take care of their physical body?
- Find a sense of meaning?
- Emotionally attune to their partner?
- Maintain their mental health?

These are just a few questions that you can use to create a vision of how you would like to experience life differently. Because your experience up to this point may be so colored with the effects of your trauma, it may be difficult to envision what a different life would actually look like. That's okay. Just do the best you can. This exercise is not about getting it right, it is about getting things going. Be sure to allow this vision to evolve as you move further down your path to recovery. You may find it helpful to go through this exercise every four to six months.

Successfully Navigating Your Journey

The most important truth that I have discovered through my personal journey of trauma recovery, as well as my clinical work helping others, is this: the people who rebuild their lives following emotional trauma are the ones who are willing to do the work of being vulnerable and taking action. Recovery doesn't happen through self-knowledge or saying the right things to yourself in the mirror. It happens through an honest and sober inventory of the parts of you that have been wounded, and a willingness to do whatever it takes to heal. The path to recovery is not simple, nor is it easy. But it can be done. I have done it. A lot of people have done it. The key is to pocket your fear and self-doubt and get busy.

I have confidence in you, and I want to hear about your success. Good luck on your journey!

Resources

I have created a page with many additional resources to help you in your healing journey. You can find them on my website at:

drtodd.com/resources

Or scan this QR code:

Index

A

acute trauma, 18-22, 29-31
accountability, 192-193
agency:
    definition of, 78-80
    and external boundaries, 140-142
    in trauma recovery, 139-144
Allen, Woody, 120
alarm response, 44, 62, 74, 98-99
    calming, 129-130
    fight as part of, 44, 100
    flight as part of, 44, 98
    freeze as part of, 44, 102
    fawn as part of, 44, 103
alcohol,
    avoiding, 151-152
anger, 49
art therapy, as therapy, 144-146
attachment, 70, 90
    adult, 91-95
    anxious, 93
    as basic instinct,
    avoidant, 93-94
    bonds, emotional, 89-91
    childhood in, 89-95
    disorganized, 94-95
    and emotional attunement,
    need for,
    secure, 92
    styles, 92-95
    trauma and, 7
attachment trauma, 22-23, 29-31
attunement, emotional,
    in relationships, 89
Automatisme psychologique, L' (Janet),
autonomic nervous system (ANS), 42-43, 62
    parasympathetic nervous system (PNS), 43
    sympathetic nervous system (SNS), 43-46

B

Blatt, Sydney, 65
boundaries,
    external, 31-33
    internal, 33-34
    setting, 140-142
Bowlby, John, 70
breathing, as therapy, 132-134
Breuer, Josef, 16-17

C

calming emotions, 12
Ceaușescu, Nicolae, 71
childhood trauma, 3
cluster of parts, 67-69
communication hygiene, 187-194
complex posttraumatic stress disorder (CPTSD), 37
core self-concept, 7, 64-65
    agency, 78-80, 182
    connection, 70-73, 180
    development of, 65-66
    healing, 12, 156

identity, 67-70, 180
trauma, effect of, 37, 63-64, 66, 80-85, 155-156
in reltionship conflict, 96-97
safety, 73-75, 181
value, 75-77, 181
crying valve, 57-58

D

Daily Recovery Journal, 173-175
depression, 3-4,
demons, personal *see* personal demons.
Diagnostic and Statistical Manual of Mental Disorders (DSM), 17
DSM-III, 17
dissociation, 55, 59-60, 70, 102
dysfunctional families, *see* relationships, dysfunctional.
dysregulation, emotional, *see* emotional dysregulation.

E

EMDR, *see* eye movement desensitization and reprocessing (EMDR).
emotional brain,
trauma, changes in, 39-40
emotional dysregulation, 5,7, 37, 49, 129
emotional flashbacks, 6, 46-47
emotional freedom technique, 138-139
emotional inflection points, 98,161-162
as therapy, 163-166
emotional neglect, 23-26, 71-73
emotional trauma, 17-18

effects of, 3, 7, 30-31, 37-38, 89-90, 115
recovery from, 12-13
relationship conflict from, 95-97
symptoms of, 9-11,46, 49, 51, 53, 55, 57, 60
emotions,
definition of, 40
primary, 185-187
secondary, 185-187
Epic of Gilgamesh, 15
epigenesis, 11
eye movement desensitization and reprocessing (EMDR), 8, 147-149

F

false fate, 117-118
fear,
in response to threat, 74
fight/flight response, *see* alarm response.
forgiveness, 125-126
Freud, Sigmund, 16-17

G

grounding, as therapy, 130-132

H

hypervigilance, *see also* trauma, hypervigilance in,
hysteria, 16-17
Freud and Breuer on, 17

I

inflection points, emotional,
see emotional inflection points.
inflection point exercise, 197-199

INDEX

internal family systems (IFS), 68

J

James, William, 16
Janet, Pierre, 16
journaling, as therapy, 142-144

L

L'automatisme Psychologique (Janet), 16
LeBanc, Mark, 117
lifestyle changes, as therapy, 149-152

M

media exposure, as triggering, 152
mirror neurons, 71

N

Napoleonic Wars, 15

P

paranoia, 51
parasympathetic nervous system (PNS), *see* autonomic nervous system, parasympathetic nervous system.
people pleasing, 6
perception,
    distorsions in, 81-82, 162-163
personal demons, 157-160
    the demon of disorientation, 158
    the demon of fear, 159
    the demon of helplessness, 159-160
    the demon of isolation, 158
    the demon of unlovability, 159
    reparenting, 172-173

physical activity:
    calming effect of,
    in trauma therapy,
Polarities of Experience (Blatt), 65
psychedelic therapy, 149
PTSD (posttraumatic stress disorder), 17
    EMDR in treatment of, 148

R

relationships:
    abusive, 35
    communication in, 178-179, 182, 194-200
    conflict in, 96-97, 112, 183-184
    disruption due to trauma, 37, 177-178
    dysfunctional, 35,
    emotional attunement in, 90-91,
    functional, 106-108
    repair in, 84-85
    strengthening, 13
    struggling, 108-110
    as therapy, 137-138
    toxic, 110-112
resentment, 125-126
Rotter, Julian, 78

S

safe space, as therapy, 136-137
safety:
    as self-concept need, 73-75
    in trauma recovery, 130-139
Schwartz, Richard, 68
self-concept, *see* core self-concept.
self-doubt, 82
self-esteem, 75-76
self-evaluation exercise, 202-211

Sexual Violence Center of Minneapolis, 2, 81
shame:
  healthy, 26
  internalized, 82, 124-125
  toxic, 26
shame-based parenting, 26-27
Shapiro, Francine, 147
social media, 152
social support, 137-138
solitary confinement, 71
Stories:
  A Fourteen-Year-Old Idiot, 47-49
  Big Mike, 103-104
  Evaporating on the Inside, 102-103
  Flooded with Rage, 28-29
  Going into Little Space, 54-55
  Her Outburst Came Out of Nowhere, 51-53
  His Late Flights, 99-100
  I Don't Know How to Pick Women, 24-26
  I Feel So Broken Inside, 35-37
  I Just Go Numb, 55-57
  I Shot My Uncle, 19-21
  Just Go Do Something, 61
  The Marine in the Hallway, 58-59
  The Masked Intruder, 21-22
  The Most Perfect Family in the World, 166-167
  Rejecting Another Relationship, 169-170
  Sitting in His Car, 101-102
  Sitting in the Audience, 60
  The Tripping Toddler, 40-41
  The Wrong Fondue, 49-51
stress,

Studies on Hysteria (Breuer and Freud), 16-17
support groups, 138
sympathetic dominance, 45-46, 62
sympathetic nervous system (SNS), *see* autonomic nervous system, sympathethic nervous system.

T

tapping, as therapy, *see also* emotional freedom technique, 138-139
trauma, *see* emotional trauma.
traumatic memory, 62, 144

V

Van der Kolk, Bessel, 148
Vietnam War, 17
vent du boulet syndrome, 15

W

Wundt, Wilhelm, 16

Y

Yoga, as therapy, 135-136

Acknowledgments

It is hard to know where to start. I feel that I am but one small voice in an ecosystem of brilliant people whose ideas have shaped my understanding of the world and whose talents have made this book possible. Although my name is on the cover, my only claim is that perhaps I am offering a slightly different perspective on a collection of work that has proceeded me. Much of my work has been heavily influenced by Susan Johnson, Les Greenberg, John Bowlby, Cindy Hazan, Philip Shaver, Bill Doherty, Eric Fromm, Bessel van der Kolk, Richard Schwartz, Judith Herman, and Francine Shapiro, as well as the founders of Alcoholics Anonymous, Bill Wilson and Dr. Bob Smith.

I would like to thank Dr. Kurt Wical, the co-founder of the Minnesota Couple Therapy Center, whose combination of compassion, leadership, generosity, and ninja-level clinical skills has profoundly impacted my clinical work, as well as the clients I have worked with over the years who have taught me more about myself than any textbook or therapist. I would also like to acknowledge the many men and women who helped me heal during my own journey of recovery.

This book would not be possible without the hard work of many talented people—first and foremost is my wife, Monique, who endured countless hours of proofreading drafts as well as my good friend and colleague Danielle Reeve for her valuable insights. My editors, Katherine Pickett of POP Editorial Services, and Sandy Wendel of Write On Inc. were invaluable in helping to shape and clean up the content of the book.

I would also like to thank all of the readers who provided valuable feedback during the preparation of the manuscript: Chip Neuenschwander, Diana Johnson, and all of the beta readers who provided me with volumes of valuable feedback.

Most importantly, I would like to thank you for reading this book. All of this work would have been for nothing if no one read it. I appreciate your interest in what I have to say, and I hope that you will find value in this work.

About the Author

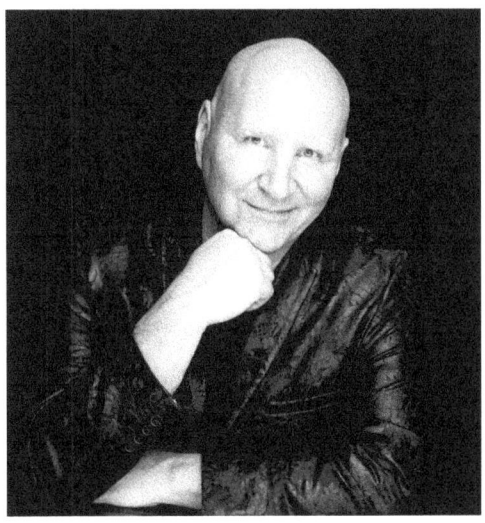

Dr. Todd Berntson is a Minnesota-based therapist, coach, and author who specializes in trauma, emotional attachment, and relationships. Best known for his practical, skills-based approach to emotional communication and healing, he has helped thousands of people live happier lives through his clinical work, workshops, and media. He is the author of the new book *Recovering from Emotional Trauma: Essential Tools to Calm Your Emotions, Heal Your Sense of Self, and Strengthen Relationships*, and can be found online at his *Dr. Todd* YouTube channel and *The Happy Neurotics Podcast*.

You can visit his website at: drtodd.com

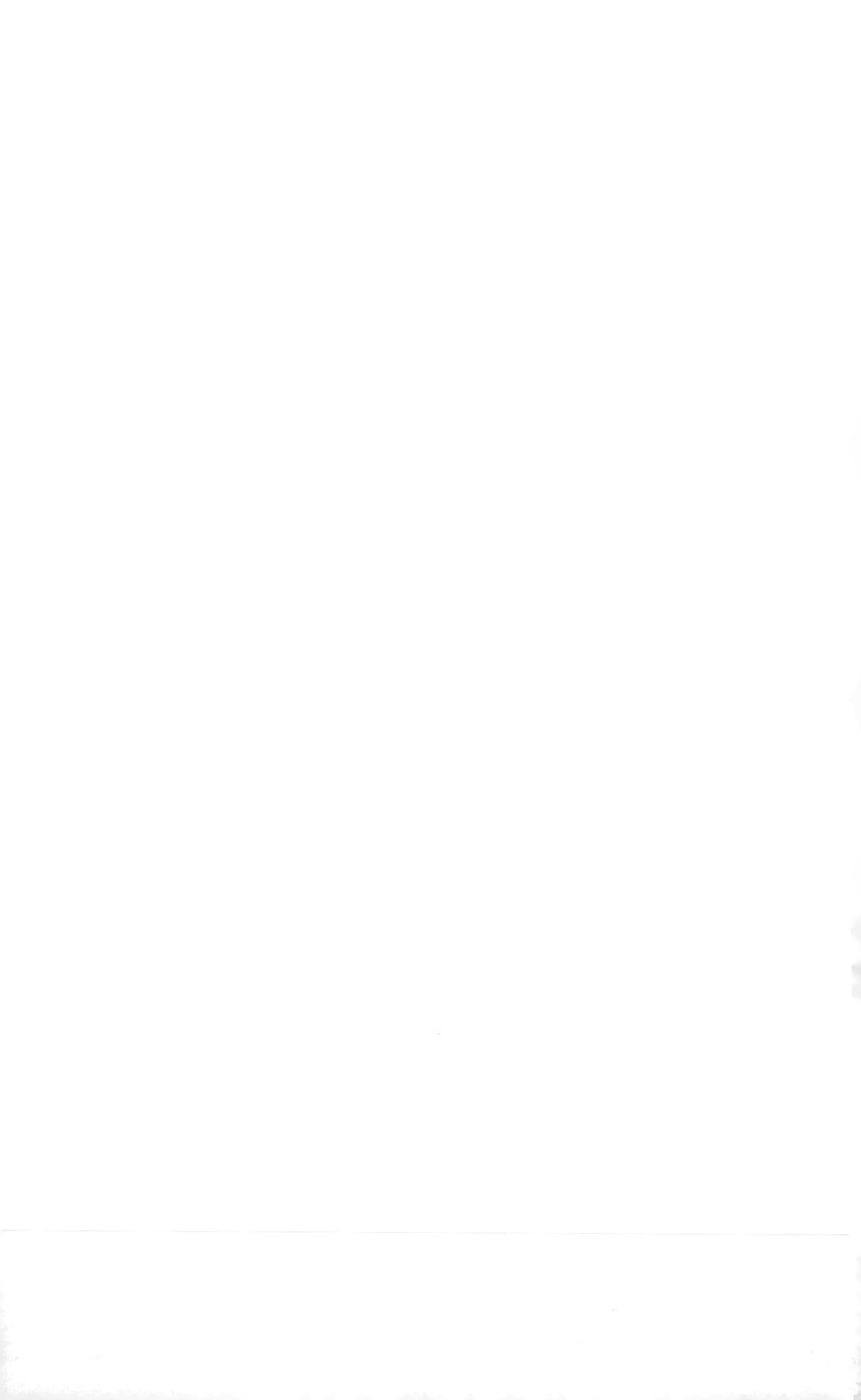

www.ingramcontent.com/pod-product-compliance
Ingram Content Group UK Ltd.
Pitfield, Milton Keynes, MK11 3LW, UK
UKHW021519120825
461708UK00001B/2